The Lost Weight Workshop

The Lost Weight Workshop

DOING THE "DIET THING" DIFFERENTLY

Karen Imhof

Cover Design by Rannee Angeli Rojo
Author Photograph by Lauren Imhof
ISBN-13: 9781517483524

ISBN-10: 1517483522

CreateSpace Independent Publishing Platform
North Charleston, South Carolina

Contents

In loving memory of my dear colleague, Lisa Linton-Farver. Your joy was contagious and your love abounded. Oh, how I imagine the heavens filled with your stories, as tears of laughter stream down the face of God. Your love and passion have left a forever imprint on this world.

Acknowledgements

~

I AM TRULY GRATEFUL FOR my wonderful family and friends who have supported me in the writing and publishing of *The Lost Weight Workshop*. Your encouragement and expertise have helped bring this book to completion. Many thanks go to:

My son, Gabriel, who bears the blame for this crazy endeavor. The night you returned from college and encouraged me to finish this book set into motion an unexpected writing frenzy. Without you, this book would quite possibly fail to exist. Thank you for letting God speak through you.

My dear friend, Tammy Gingras-Moore, who faithfully offered encouragement throughout the writing process and believed that the message of *The Lost Weight Workshop* needed to be shared.

My prayer circle: Jean Snyder, Sharon Zehr, Tina Barnhart, Tina Bender and Kathy Neff. I know your prayers have already impacted future readers of this book.

My Mama Kathy Neff. You have always believed in me, and I am forever grateful.

My editors, Jeannette Dilouie (JDiLouie@innovativeediting.com) and Kristen Staley (writerkms@aol.com). Your insights and expertise were invaluable to this project.

My children, Gabe, Liz, Josh and Lauren. You are the light of my world and the joy in my heart. Oh, how you make me smile!

My husband, John, for all of your love and support. I wouldn't have wanted to do it without you.

My Heavenly Father, who has given me vision and a voice to share with many. Thank you for loving me so lavishly that you sent your son to die for me. I know you will never leave me nor forsake me. You are my rock, my strong tower and my fortress. You truly are my everything!

Author's Note

I IMAGINE YOU'VE PURCHASED THIS book with the hope of a fresh start. A new beginning. But the voice of fear speaks loud and clear, prompting you to wonder…

"Will it really be different this time? I have failed at 'this diet thing' so many times."

The answer is yes! It will be different because the Lost Weight Workshop is different. Here's why: Instead of striving to lose weight, you will be resting in God's promises of victory. Your motivation will originate from a vision of a spectacular life rather than obtaining a lower number on the scale, and your health will become a gift you open daily instead of a list of to-dos to achieve.

The Lost Weight Workshop has been birthed from my personal story of addiction to food and dieting. My battle with compulsive eating began at the age of eleven and continued into my early twenties. Through dieting, I learned to sneak food, binge and of course, hide the evidence. Sugar was my friend, my enemy, my drug of choice. I was consumed with losing weight, and I struggled with the battle that raged inside me to not eat the foods "forbidden" by my diet.

When I gave into my binges, the aftermath was devastating; the waves of guilt and shame followed by the overwhelming fear of starting yet another diet and failing, or of taking a bite of food and all hell breaking loose. After successfully following a Christian weight loss program, I was convinced I would never binge again. But I was wrong. I came home from college one weekend and took a spoonful of peanut butter; and that one bite set off a month-long binge. I ate myself to a sickening fullness each night, rationalizing that I would start my diet tomorrow. But each tomorrow only brought more of the same destructive cycle.

If the physical and emotional toll of what I have described above resonates with you, keep reading and don't give up.

You may feel as though life has passed you by due to the choices you've made, but God provides a fresh beginning every morning filled with His mercy and love (Lamentations 3:22-23). You can choose to remain paralyzed in your circumstances created by life's adversities, or you can opt to shift the direction of your life by embracing the truth of God's love for you. You can wallow in the reality of being overweight, or you can celebrate in the fact that you are a child of God entitled to all His promises.

You do not have to walk as a victim of your circumstances any longer.

Refuse to believe that it's too late, that you're not worth it or that you've failed too many times, for these are lies of defeat. Even if you don't feel strong enough to embrace change for yourself, remember that it is not in your strength that you will conquer. It is in His (2 Corinthians 12:9-11).

Let's approach dieting and weight loss differently, and get off the merry-go-round. Let's stop aligning ourselves with a dieting system that promises an emotional rollercoaster of guilt, fear and failure. Instead, let's embrace God's promises of peace, vision and victory. Don't settle any longer. Dream with great expectation, and experience the beauty God has for your life!

Blessings,

Karen (Mama K) Imhof

Week One

~

WELCOME TO THE LOST WEIGHT WORKSHOP!

THE LOST WEIGHT WORKSHOP (LWW) is designed to help you do the "diet thing" differently by shedding truth on the misconceptions of dieting, while equipping you with tools to break free from the dieting cycle. You will find yourself stretched to step out of your comfort zone and to look at the dieting structure from a new perspective: a perspective that may challenge what you've always believed or done in the past. If you are reading this book, I would bet that what you've done in the past has not yielded lasting results. So what do you have to lose? I ask you to ponder the truths of the LWW, not as an observer or for knowledge's sake, but with the goal to explore, question and contemplate them. Expect to discover something new as God reveals His promises to you.

BEFORE YOU GET STARTED

1. **Buy a journal.**

Journaling is an important piece of the LWW. You will want to purchase a journal or use the pages provided at the end of each chapter. If you merely read without taking the time to explore the journal sections, you will walk away with increased knowledge but little else. Don't rush the process. You may find yourself rereading a chapter because God is speaking to you from that specific section. You are on a marvelous journey of discovery; soak it in, and remember that what you discover along the way will yield greater value and impact than the goal of reaching the finish line.

I've also provided a tracker for the day-to-day journey, which is located in Appendix A. As you use it, you will be encouraged to focus each day on what is important: time with God, the gifts of health and a heart of praise. Some of the concepts used in the tracker are clearly explained as you progress throughout the book, but it should not prevent you from using it beginning in Week One.

A word of caution: If after reading Week One, you find that you strongly identify with the dieter's mentality, I would recommend that you do *not* use the tracker until Week Eight. The concern is that you will use it as a limiting dieting tool, reinforcing the behaviors of the dieting cycle. Instead, give yourself time to soak in the newness of what God is doing.

2. **Keep asking the question.**

As you read *The Lost Weight Workshop*, you'll want to keep the following questions at the forefront of your mind: "What am I aligning myself with, and is it producing the kind of fruit I want in my life?" *Webster's Dictionary* defines align this way: "to get into line, to change (something) so that it agrees with or matches something else."[1]

Imagine yourself hiking through the mountains and being faced with two different paths ahead. On one path, you will cross under a waterfall; the other, you will travel under a rockslide. Depending on your decision, you will either get soaking wet or knocked in the head. The reason for this outcome is based on this simple principle of alignment: You "got in line" with one of the above options. And the one you chose determined the result: being refreshed or all banged up.

Throughout our lifetime, we are presented with opportunities to align with people, events, activities and *beliefs* that have a direct impact on our overall well-being. And our choices determine the level of truth or toxicity that flows in and out of our lives, creating a residual effect not only on ourselves but for those around us as well.

There is a reason why God says, "Whatever things are true, whatever things are noble, whatever things are just, whatever things are pure, whatever things are lovely, whatever things are of good report, if there is any virtue and if there is anything praiseworthy – meditate on these things" (Philippians 4:8). He knows that what you choose to focus your thoughts on will produce either a positive or negative chain reaction in your life.

Learning how to do the diet thing differently will happen as we first identify and turn away from the thoughts and patterns we have aligned with that keep us tied to the dieting cycle, and then choose to "get in line" with God's promises. As you read, keep asking yourself the questions of: *What am I aligning myself with?* and *Is it producing the kind of fruit I want in my life?* Stay open-minded as God reveals the answers.

3. Let God break up the fallow ground of your heart.

My youngest daughter loves to garden. Each spring, she prepares her garden with great anticipation of the delicious vegetables she will grow. Her excitement tends to waiver as she carefully works to prepare the soil, but she remains committed knowing that – without the necessary effort of digging up the soil, weeding and watering her plants – she won't enjoy the fruit of her labor: her red juicy tomatoes.

Personally, I don't enjoy gardening. Getting dirty, digging up the ground, and spending time to weed and water isn't my idea of relaxation and fun. But I know that, if I want to eat fresh tomatoes from the garden, then I (or thankfully, my daughter or husband) must devote the necessary effort to prepare the soil. Planting a garden takes time and an abundance of love devoted to the daily tasks; it is not merely a plant-it-and-leave-it process.

The weight loss journey is no different. It takes time and heaps of love!

In Jeremiah 4:3, God says to break up the unplowed ground of our hearts and to not sow our seed among thorns. Just like the sower of the parable in Matthew 13, if we don't break up the fallow ground of our hearts before embracing the weight loss journey, comfortable and familiar habits, the stress of life or the issues of the heart will rise up to choke out the hope of shedding our unwanted weight. This is the reason that, *prior* to embarking on the weight loss journey, *The Lost Weight Workshop* focuses on aligning our hearts, renewing our beliefs and healing the emotional ties to food.

When we make the decision to lose weight, we tend to plunge full steam ahead, racing to buy the newest diet book, signing up for the latest weight loss program, joining a gym, and buying a new outfit one size smaller while visualizing ourselves wearing it.

Whew! Sounds exhausting!

I know that the anticipation of losing weight or fitting into a new dress or pant size is thrilling, much like the first fruits of the garden. You may be tempted to skip the preparation stage, eager to jump right in. But if you do, you will only find yourself riding on the same dieting rollercoaster, once again feeling frustrated and dismayed with the results.

As you begin this incredible journey, you will discover it's a dirty process to dig up the issues that have kept you bound to the losing-and-gaining cycle. Your heart may be messy because – let's face it – life is messy. To do this diet thing differently, you will spend time weeding out your old beliefs about dieting and watering your soul with God's promises. The work you put into preparing your heart and mind will be well worth the investment; not only will you lose your unwanted pounds, but you will reap a peaceful relationship with food and ultimate freedom from the dieting cycle.

My daughter's tomatoes are the fruit of her labor of love in preparing and tending her garden; and you too will reap a harvest from your labor of love that goes far beyond weight loss. Devote the time required to prepare your heart; you will yield different results. You will reap a beautiful harvest.

JOURNAL

As you prepare for this journey, give God permission to break up the fallow ground of your heart. God is a gentleman; He won't barge in and start digging unless you ask Him to. You must be brave enough to ask. Allow Him to lovingly begin the process of revealing what keeps your heart connected to the vicious cycle of gaining and losing. It might be messy, yes, but what beauty will be harvested!

Below is a sample prayer, but I encourage you to write your own. Speak to God from your heart, and express your deepest thoughts and desires to Him.

Dear God,

I am ready to do this "diet thing" differently. Help me see and understand what keeps me bound to the dieting cycle, and I ask you to gently plow up the parts of my heart that keep me from experiencing all that you have for me. Set me free, God! I accept the freedom and healing that you have for me. I will not fear the unknown. I will no longer let the past dictate the life I live. I welcome your wisdom and I embrace change. Thank you for your awesome love that will take me though this journey.

Now that you have a journal, are prepared to answer the questions of alignment and have given God permission to dig up the unplowed ground of your heart, you are equipped to begin the discovery of doing the "diet thing" differently. Enjoy the journey!

JOURNAL NOTES

_____

_____

_____

_____

_____

_____

_____

_____

_____

_____

_____

_____

_____

_____

_____

_____

_____

_____

_____

_____

_____

_____

_____

_____

_____

_____

_____

~♪

CHAPTER 2

Dissecting the Dieting Process

WE HAVE PROBABLY ALL HEARD the saying that "diets don't work," and most of us would agree; yet when we find ourselves with excess weight to lose, what course of action do we take? We go on a diet. So why do we continue to diet when we recognize they don't work? Is there a different way to go about attacking the issue of weight loss?

This week, we'll be dissecting the dieting process to discover the answer to the question of why you should do the "diet thing" differently. Because we are taking a magnifying glass to the flawed system of dieting, it may feel a bit tedious. But we need to make sense of why diets do not work before we can understand how to proceed. Once we've taken things apart, we will begin rebuilding – this time from God's beginning point and upon His foundation. As you read, ask God to reveal how you have aligned with the dieting structure and in what ways it has impacted you.

Diets Have a Low Success Rate

Over twenty years ago when I worked as a weight management counselor, the quoted success rate for an individual who dieted, lost weight and kept the pounds off was about 5%. Even though studies are showing a wider range of success (2%-20%), the truth is that the obesity rate in America is not declining, and diet and health programs are not solving this epidemic.[1,2]

A question worth pondering is this: Why do we continue to subscribe to something that guarantees such a high potential for failure? If you were presented with the opportunity to invest your time, energy and money into a business venture with a 95% chance of failing, would you do it? Business savvy or not, you would certainly be smart enough to turn down the investment opportunity.

Diets Are Costly

Years ago, as I was spending time with God, He asked, "What if you never thought about your weight again?" My response: "Wow, how freeing that would be. I would have so much time on my hands, mentally and emotionally. And, of course, more money to spend."

The weight loss journey involves a significant investment. We financially invest in the newest diet books, weight loss meetings, health programs and unused gym memberships. Gym memberships are a worthwhile expense if we actually go to the gym. I finally decided that I wouldn't buy another health or diet book unless I felt God prompting me to, because I already owned a plethora of them, which were already collecting dust on a shelf. No need to continue to spend money on unnecessary diet books when I could be investing my money more wisely.

Not only do we invest financially, but we spend an exorbitant amount of time mentally fixating on the weight loss process. When we start a new diet, our day is spent thinking about the food we are eating or not eating, if we've lost or gained weight, how our clothes are fitting, whether we are satisfied or not with what we see reflected in the mirror, whether we've been "good" on our diet, etc.

Not only do we invest our money and mental energy, but one of the greatest sacrifices made involves the emotional expense. Each time we embark on a new diet, we begin with the hope and dream of losing weight; but as we experience another round of unsuccessful dieting, we take a ride on the emotional rollercoaster with a multitude of feelings ranging from disappointment to utter despair. In my early years of dieting, the emotional investment took the greatest toll. My self-esteem was wrapped around being thin; and every time I failed, I was engulfed in the destructive emotional cycle of guilt, condemnation and self-hatred.

So why do we, as intelligent people, continue to follow a dieting process that requires such a high level of investment yet promises such a low success rate?

DIETS ARE A SHORTSIGHTED GOAL

The standard course of action when we need to lose weight is to go on a diet. If we're one of the lucky few to actually reach our weight loss goal, what happens next? *We have reached the finish line. We have conquered and won.* But is the accomplishment of achieving the prize of weight loss strong enough to hold us to our desired number on the scale? Or, over time, do we revert back to former eating habits and a busy life where exercise becomes a distant wish? Before we know it, does the weight we lost find its way home with a few additional pounds?

Losing weight feels good in the moment, but rarely is it a strong enough motivator to keep up with the larger investment. Why? Because it's a short-term, temporary goal that, once accomplished, does not sustain lasting results. When we diet, we set a goal. We achieve the goal, and then we are done. But achieving good health is not a short-term accomplishment. The motivation to lose weight will need to come from a purpose that has a far greater impact beyond the temporary fix of shedding pounds. If we make weight loss the target, we will continue losing and gaining, evading our desired objective for permanent and sustainable weight loss. The past is a pretty accurate and consistent indicator of what will happen in the future unless we make a change.

In my personal life, I have experienced this shortsighted cycle. I found myself with twenty unwanted pounds after a significantly rough patch of life. Three separate times, I lost the extra weight by participating in a gym competition, joining a weight-management program or designing my own guidelines. Each time, I followed the plan, exercised and succeeded. I accomplished my goal of weight loss; but after I reached the finish line, "life" would happen, as it always seems to do. A major life change would occur, the holidays would hit or a stressful situation would arise, and slowly but surely, the lost pounds would return. I realized that setting weight loss as the desired outcome yielded a temporary and shortsighted result. The thrill of losing the weight, looking better in my clothes, even having more energy, was not enough to keep up with sustaining the goal of permanent weight loss.

If we continue to set the quick fix of weight loss as the focal point of our health journey, we will fail. God wants our motivation to be healthy to originate from a life of vision and purpose rather than the physical goal of weight loss. In Week Seven, we will discover how to exchange the shortsighted goal of dieting to one with eternal significance (2 Corinthians 4:18).

Diets Are One-Dimensional

The reasons for dieting vary, from wanting to fit into a smaller pair of jeans to looking good in our summer clothes or losing our belly fat; or they may be health related, such as lowering our cholesterol or gaining more energy. Whatever the desired goal, our true motivation usually is directed towards one central target: changing our physical appearance.

Here is an essential question to ask: "Is the reason we are overweight solely limited to a physical issue?" If being fat was merely about eating too much food, than we would go on a diet, lose the weight and keep it off for life, right? In theory, yes, and we would love for it to be that simple. However, the truth is that our weight problems cannot be isolated to only the physical; it is more complicated than that because, as human beings, our design is not limited to the body. God created humans with a spirit, soul (emotions, mind and will) and body (1 Thessalonians 5:23). In trying to alter only the physical through dieting, we disregard two-thirds of who we are.

To isolate the physical from the rest of our being would be like trying to put together a puzzle with only a third of the pieces, still believing that the end result will yield a completed puzzle. Puzzle pieces are interconnected, and each one is essential to create a complete picture. We too, as beautifully designed human beings, have interconnected pieces of spirit, soul and body.

If we simply address physical change without incorporating the emotional and spiritual part of our being, than we will have intermittent change with limited success. There will be pieces of the weight loss puzzle missing that are necessary to complete our picture of health and beauty. As a result, we remain frustrated and plagued by numerous failed dieting attempts. For our weight loss journey to be successful, we must incorporate all of our being: spirit, soul and body.

DIETS CREATE AN UNHEALTHY RELATIONSHIP WITH FOOD

On most diet plans, food is lumped into categories of what we either can or cannot eat: good vs. bad. There are inherent problems with this "can't have" mentality. Diets that restrict foods put us in a state of self-denial, which can result in an unhealthy desire for – or even an obsession with – food. What happens within human nature when we're told we can't have something we want? What happens when we follow a diet plan that forbids a certain food? Our self-indulgent behavior takes over and we shout back, "BUT I WANT IT!" All we can think about is how much we really want to eat that scrumptious treat. The food begins to mock us from the refrigerator, calling our name. We can think of nothing else. I know from experience that some foods have an audible voice.

Adam and Eve are the perfect example of how human nature wants what it cannot have. When God instructed them to not eat the fruit from the "Tree of Knowledge of Good and Evil," what did Satan use to tempt them? The fruit they were forbidden to eat (Genesis 3:1-7). If Adam and Eve could not successfully manage the "can't haves" in their perfect environment with God, why do we believe we are going to be any more successful in our imperfect world with our flawed lives? Living in a state of self-denial is an unrealistic approach to creating a healthy relationship with food.

Furthermore, dieting ignites irrational thinking in relationship to food. When we eat a forbidden food, we can adopt an "I've blown it" philosophy. Simply put, since we've already blown our diet, we might as well really blow it. We will deliberately "cheat" on our diet: One cookie becomes the whole pack or a few French fries morph into an oversized value meal. Can you imagine yourself advising a friend to eat an entire bag of potato chips just because she ate something that wasn't on her diet? Ridiculous! Right? Yet we do this to ourselves all in the name of dieting.

DIETS ARE BASED IN PERFORMANCE AND PERFECTION

Diets tell us what to eat, how much to eat, what not to eat and sometimes even when to eat. In the beginning, we diligently follow the plan set before us. If we have what we would deem a successful diet week – meaning we perfectly adhered to the plan – then we are happy. All is well. But if we do not have a victorious diet week, consuming foods that are prohibited, than we feel guilty. We're reluctant to step on the scale or attend our weight loss meeting, all because we fear what the scale will reveal.

And God forbid if we've been "perfect" following our diet and the scale shows our weight has INCREASED. Then all is really not well! We feel frustrated and angry. In fact, anyone in the near vicinity should run for cover. I have overheard women say they wanted to throw the scale out the window when they had a "perfect" week and yet their weight still increased.

When that happens, what do we do? We retaliate with a "punish the scale" attitude: "Oh yeah? I'll show you! I'll eat those gooey chocolate brownies I baked for my kids! Which, by the way, I didn't even lick the spoon when preparing them because I WAS BEING PERFECT ON MY DIET!" Under this type of mentality, we may find ourselves leaving our weight loss meeting and driving straight to the drive-thru window, all because the scale did not reflect our expectation of our perfect performance. And so we completely sabotage any chance of success.

Depending on the magnitude of the relationship between our weight and self-esteem, we may also experience a deeper emotional response to this performance and perfection mentality. There is a point during the dieting process where we perform for a season, following the plan and denying ourselves, but the day inevitably arrives when we grow weary of trying to be perfect. Temptation calls and we give in. Or rather, we give up. As the magnetic pull of the foods we've avoided for weeks begins to increase, we can no longer resist. When those foods deemed off-limits eventually reach our lips, we experience a euphoric sensation. One bite leads to two, and two leads to three, until we have stuffed ourselves beyond full.

It tastes so good while it's going down, but as we come to the end of the drug-like experience, all-consuming thoughts of regret and guilt begin to surface. Along with condemnation, waves of fear and anxiety rise up, especially for those of us who have previously experienced this behavior. We fear that we will start gaining weight; we fear we won't be able to get "back on" our diet.

As panic and anxiety engulf our emotions, our thoughts become even more focused on food. We begin spiraling out of control as the mental battle takes hold. "I shouldn't eat that. I can't have it, but I want it." As the battle rages on, we become obsessed with thoughts of food and overcome with waves of regret; peace is nowhere to be found. The cycle of performance/perfection has won. We spiral to a place of hopelessness believing: "I've failed again. I will never lose this weight."

As we find ourselves trapped in this destructive cycle:

* We are overwhelmed with discouragement.
* We eat.
* We become immersed with guilt and condemnation.
* We eat.
* We are inundated with fear and anxiety.
* We eat.
* We start a new diet.
* We perform perfectly for a time.
* We fail.
* We eat.
* We are buried in hopelessness.
* We eat... and the cycle continues.

Again, I have to ask: Why would intelligent human beings buy into a system that produces such irrational behavior? Why do we accept this process as normal?

~⁀

CHAPTER 3

My Dieting Cycle

I EXPERIENCED THIS DESTRUCTIVE CYCLE during a twelve-year period of my life. My weight loss journey began around the age of eleven, when I was in sixth grade. My friends were petite and had not yet hit puberty. I, on the other hand, was already physically maturing and a head taller than both the boys and girls. When my friends were wearing training bras, I was wearing a size 32D. I was five-foot three-inches and weighed 118 pounds; not what you would call overweight, but I felt different and was heavy in my eyes.

My sweet mom handled my situation using the knowledge she had gathered from her own personal struggles with food and dieting. And together, we joined a well-known weight management program. I don't recall if I actually lost any weight; I only know that it was the start of what I label as my twelve-year dieting career. I could not tell you a time during that period where dieting, food and my weight were not the obsessions of my life.

My world for those years evolved around diets of all types, some healthy and some quite extreme: the rice diet, a liquid cherry diet (which was quite gross), Christian programs, non-Christian programs… You name it, I probably tried it. I was addicted to the dieting process, the desire to be thin and the compliments from others that accompanied my weight loss. My self-esteem was directly connected to my physical appearance; and in my eyes, my body was never thin enough or pretty enough. I was consumed with feelings of failure and self-hatred. Even though I was never obese, in my mind, 10 pounds or 100 pounds of extra weight hardly mattered because it all added up to being fat and unacceptable.

I learned a great deal from the dieting process, not much of which I would call positive. The most detrimental and life-altering lesson was the art of sneaking and binging on what I deemed to be the "can't have" foods. Instead of eating a candy bar and enjoying it, I would go to the grocery store, buy three or four, consume them all on the drive home and hide the evidence…all under the guise of dieting.

This behavior created a vicious cycle of binging, guilt and shame. When I ate the "can't have" foods, it fueled my craving for them. I would feel guilty, fueling my desire to eat more, which led to intense waves of remorse and regret. What an emotionally draining cycle! Each summer, I would dream of going to fat camp so I could be thin and stop the madness. I didn't know what it felt like to be an alcoholic, but I remember thinking that compulsive eating was an addiction that no one seemed to be discussing.

My compulsive eating behavior continued throughout high school and into college. During my sophomore year of college, my addiction reached an unprecedented high. I remember going to the grocery store each night, looking for food to feed my binges. I would walk up and down the cookie aisle, buy a box of cookies, return to my sorority house and devour the entire box. Along with being overwhelmed with the usual shame and guilt, I would go to bed feeling physically sick but convinced I would begin my diet the next morning. The morning would come, but the diet would never start. Off to the store I would go; and the destructive, compulsive cycle would begin anew.

Needless to say, that was a tough semester.

My Healing Journey

My healing occurred in two phases. The first part began the summer after my first year of graduate school, as I was in the planning stages of my next diet so that I could return to school "skinny." That's when I clearly heard God say, "Do not go on a diet."

Although it wasn't an audible voice, it was a moment that caused me to stop what I was thinking and take notice. Sometimes God speaks softly with a gentle nudge; but this time, He spoke loud and clear. I was not to go on a diet.

That summer, I didn't worry about what I was eating, how much I was eating or if I was losing weight. Instead of dieting, I ate regular food and normal portions, and dinner was whatever Mom prepared. I was at peace with food and myself – not striving to lose weight.

My healing began when I said "no" to dieting, but my worth as a person was still wrapped around attaining a certain body type. My perception of my body image was completely distorted. Even to this day, I'm surprised at how completely inaccurate my mental picture was of my physical appearance.

Recently, my teenage daughter tried on one of my dresses from college, which was form-fitting with a slim, long skirt. My daughter, with her tiny waist and great little figure, had trouble getting into the dress; but when she managed to put it on, it fit perfectly. At that moment, I realized that – when I wore that dress – I would have never described myself as having a small waist or slim figure. In my mind, I always needed to lose weight.

If I was to live in complete freedom from the bondage to food and dieting, the way I saw myself in the mirror required a major transformation. I am so thankful that God continued this healing process, which began shortly after graduate school. I had moved from Oklahoma to work in Pennsylvania, and I joined a little country church that had a passion for the things of God. A core group of young adults would meet weekly for a Bible study, where we discovered that God wanted us healed and set free. As I grew closer to God, I realized that I didn't want my entire life to center on losing weight. Yet at that point, that is exactly what it consisted of: seeking thinness and the perfect body.

I remember the day I sat before God and declared that I didn't want to be standing before Him at the end of my life, facing the truth that dieting and losing weight were my sole accomplishments. That moment stands as the turning point when God radically touched my life.

Sometimes when God takes us through the healing process, it is just that: a process. Our healing usually comes through faith and diligence to stand fast as we lay hold of God's promises. But He took me on a different path. He simply set me free. One day, I looked in the mirror and hated my appearance; the next, I did not. It is much like the stories you hear of the alcoholic who is radically set free from addiction after God gets a hold of his life. One day, he drinks alcohol; the next he doesn't. No withdrawals, no side effects. Just freedom. That was my experience: free to simply be me, to be at peace with food and to love the "me" God created.

During that time, yes, I was beautifully set free from the compulsive eating cycle and hatred of my physical appearance. But my health journey still continues today with periods of highs and lows, successes and failures. As I continue on this quest, I am even more convinced that the fundamental core of the dieting process promotes unhealthy beliefs and irrational thinking. When we align ourselves with this process, with its poor success rate, lack of dimension and unhealthy relationship to food, we can expect an outpouring from the dieting belief system into our own.

Now let's take a look at how the dieting promises compare to God's promises. Don't skip over this part. If you take time to contemplate the differences, you will be amazed.

COMPARING PROMISES

1. Diets promote a low success rate.

But God promises that we are more than conquerors and that we have the victory in Him (Romans 8:37-39, 1Corinthians 15:57).

He says that all things are possible, and that we can do all things in Christ (Philippians 4:13).

2. Diets are one dimensional, only targeting the physical.

But God has designed us spirit, soul and body (1 Thessalonians 5:23).

3. The dieter's mentality produces guilt and shame.

But God says there is no condemnation for those that love him and are called according to His purpose (Romans 8:1, 8:28).

4. The dieter's mentality brings fear and anxiety.

But God says we have not been given a spirit of fear but of love, power and a sound mind (2 Timothy 1:7).

5. The dieter's mentality promotes a negative approach to food.

But with God, there is freedom. All things are permissible, but not all things are beneficial (2 Corinthians 3:17, 1 Corinthians 10:23 NIV).

6. Diets are based on performance and perfection.

But God's system is based on grace (Ephesians 2:8).

We are saved by grace, not perfection. If God had made living a perfect life and performing good deeds the criteria for getting into Heaven, than none of us would make it there. We as humans are not perfect, but God is; that's why He sent His son Jesus as a sacrifice for our imperfections. Because of this sacrificial love that God has for us, we can now live a life forgiven, at peace to know that we are loved without the compulsion to be perfect.

So if God's original plan is based on grace, why are we aligning ourselves with a system that is wholeheartedly designed around performance and perfection?

The following diagram shows what is deposited into our lives depending on our decision to align with the promises of God or those of dieting.

Aligning Our Hearts with the...

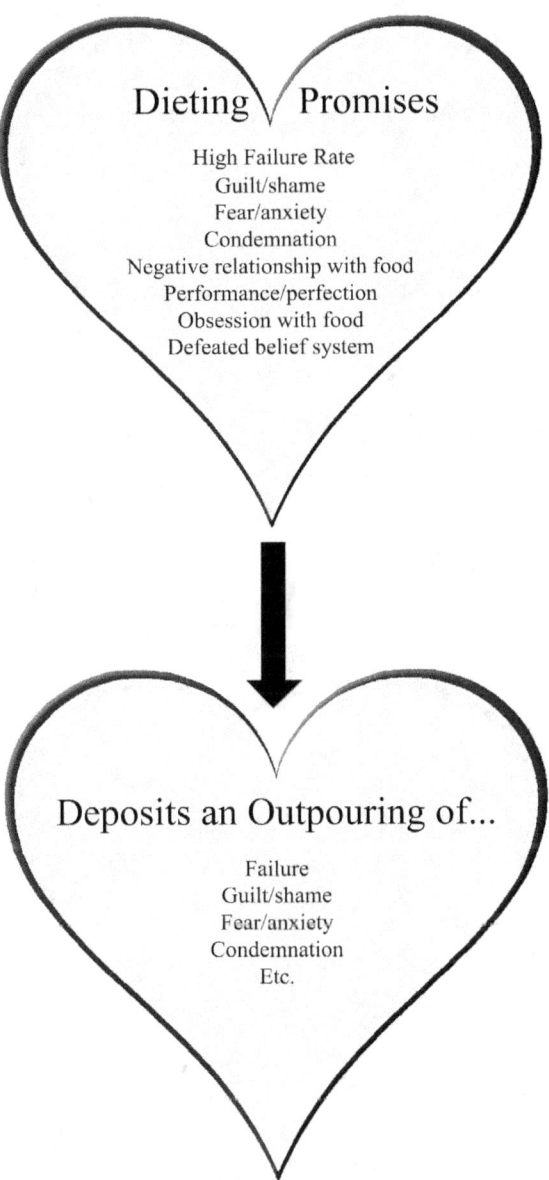

Dieting \ Promises

High Failure Rate
Guilt/shame
Fear/anxiety
Condemnation
Negative relationship with food
Performance/perfection
Obsession with food
Defeated belief system

Deposits an Outpouring of...

Failure
Guilt/shame
Fear/anxiety
Condemnation
Etc.

Keeping Us Bound to the Dieting Cycle

Aligning Our Hearts with...

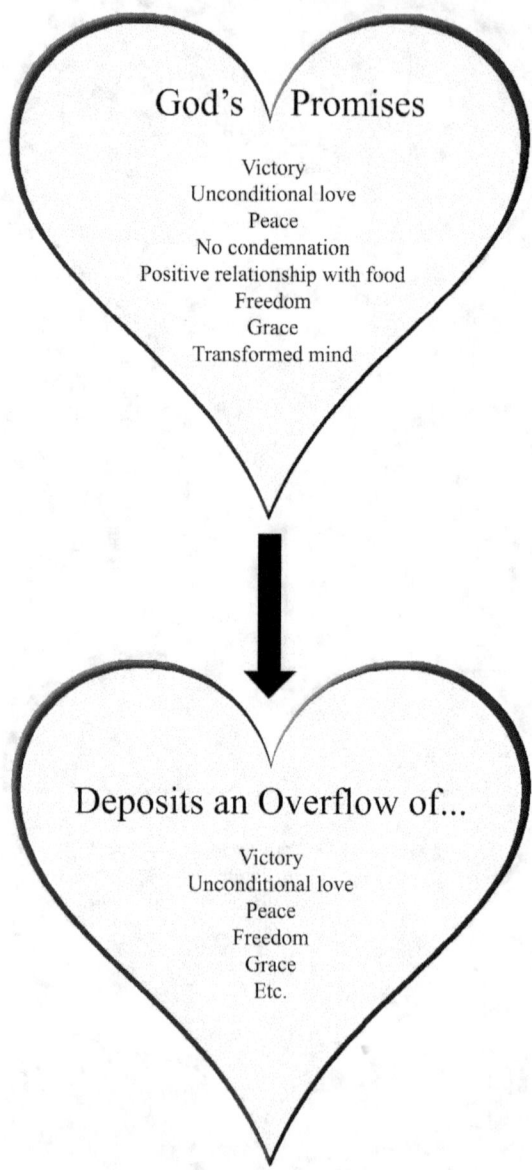

God's \ Promises

Victory
Unconditional love
Peace
No condemnation
Positive relationship with food
Freedom
Grace
Transformed mind

Deposits an Overflow of...

Victory
Unconditional love
Peace
Freedom
Grace
Etc.

Setting Us Free to Live in Victory

When you compare the promises we receive from the dieter's heart with what flows from God's heart, you can see they yield radically different outcomes. In fact, they are the exact *opposite*. We do have a choice. We can opt to align ourselves with a system fraught with a high failure rate, guilt, shame, fear, anxiety, condemnation, a negative relationship and obsession with food, performance/perfection, anxiety and defeated beliefs. Or we can choose to align with the promises of victory, unconditional love, peace, no condemnation, a positive relationship with food, freedom, grace and a transformed mind. For me, the choice is clear; I sincerely hope this is true for you as well.

Much of what I'm dissecting about the dieting system is a mindset: a belief system based on irrational thinking and behavior. You will want to assess your mental and emotional connection to the dieting process.

For those of us who have dieted and failed in a continual pattern, we relate all too well to this unhealthy process. Whether you identify strongly with the dieter's mindset or not, I hope we can all agree that the system we've been given to promote sustainable weight loss has turned out miserably for most. My hope is that, through the Lost Weight Workshop, we will do the "diet thing" differently by aligning our beliefs – not on an outdated approach – but instead on renewed thinking and behaviors that will transform not only our physical body, but our entire being: body, soul and spirit.

JOURNAL

Which would you rather have flow into your life: the promises of the dieting system or the promises of God? Ask God to specifically reveal the areas of the dieting process that you have bought into. Journal what God reveals to you. If you see yourself operating in the dieter's promises, recognize them for what they are: counterfeit and radically opposite beliefs from God's Word. Write a declaration that you will choose to align yourself with God's heart and will no longer "get in line with" the empty promises of the dieting system.

Look up each of the Scriptures on page 23. Write them in your journal, and contemplate on how life-giving they are and contradictory to the promises of dieting. Mediate on them until you believe them and accept them as your truth. Then, when you once again find yourself operating in the familiar belief patterns of performance/perfection, guilt and condemnation, you will be able to recognize them for what they are – which is FALSE – and accept the truth of God's grace and victory!

This week, when you find yourself dwelling on your weight and dieting, instead shift your thinking to align with God's promises. Your dieter's mind will be anxious to lose weight, and you will be tempted to let it take over. Remind yourself that doing the diet thing differently means changing the way you have typically approached weight loss. It will feel different, and yes, you will want to gravitate towards the way you behaved in the past.

The practice of alignment is not a one-shot deal. You will find yourself oscillating from a diet mentality to the new way of thinking about the dieting process. As you recognize yourself operating in your former beliefs, return to the promises of God and meditate on them. Allow God the opportunity to show you a different way based upon His heart and perspective.

Make this prayer your heart's desire:

Dear God,

Thank You for opening the eyes of my heart to Your truth about dieting. Forgive me for accepting the promises of a high failure rate and an unhealthy relationship with food over Your promises of victory and peace. I declare that I will no longer accept a counterfeit belief system as my reality, but I will get in line and affiliate myself with Your truth. Thank You for showing me where I have operated, and still do operate, in the dieter's belief system. I ask You to transform these areas with Your love. I will take the time to discover Your truth and will reject the old yet familiar way of thinking about the weight loss journey. Thank You that Your promises come with a God-approved guarantee to accomplish infinitely more than I might ask or imagine (Ephesians 3:20 NLT). Lord, You and Your ways are so awesome!

THOUGHTS TO PONDER AS YOU JOURNAL

1. Take a quick inventory of your thoughts toward the dieting process. Identify the parts that do not produce life. Meditate on Philippians 4:8.
2. Read Jeremiah 4:3. Pray and ask God to break up the unplowed ground of your heart. As you pray, ask Him to identify the unknown parts of your heart that keep you tied to the dieting cycle.
3. Describe your relationship with food (e.g., self-denial, I've-blown-it mentality, performance/perfection behavior).
4. What is your response to the destructive cycle of performance and perfection?

JOURNAL NOTES

_____

_____

_____

_____

_____

_____

_____

_____

_____

_____

_____

_____

_____

_____

_____

_____

_____

_____

_____

_____

_____

_____

_____

_____

_____
_____
_____
_____
_____
_____
_____
_____
_____
_____
_____
_____
_____
_____
_____
_____
_____
_____
_____
_____
_____
_____
_____
_____

Week Two

CHAPTER 4

⌒⌐

At the Starting Line

"God does not see as man sees, for man sees the outward appearance, but God sees the heart."

— *1 Samuel 16:7*

When we look at our appearance in the mirror, what do we see? Usually, our attention is drawn to all of our physical imperfections: whether we have short legs, crooked teeth, round faces or big noses… and of course, how much weight we need to lose. It's natural to focus on the physical shortcomings because we live in a world that assigns value to the outward appearance.

Likewise, growing old gracefully does not have the same implication it did a few decades ago. Today, aging means no grey hair, wrinkles, sagging skin, fat or cellulite, but a perfect smile filled with pearly white teeth. Our society is obsessed with physical perfection. We admire and idolize those who look ten to twenty years younger than their natural age; it's regarded with the same awe as winning an award or achieving something of significance.

The media has driven these unrealistic expectations for physical perfection. Years ago, advertisers used photo techniques to "enhance" the natural beauty of models; but today, instead of merely touching up photos for minor imperfections, pictures are distorted to such lengths that it's physically impossible for a human being to achieve the created image. The byproduct of this distortion is that we have generations of young people growing up believing that what they see in the media is the expected standard for physical beauty: a benchmark based upon a fabricated image. These unattainable expectations were my gauge for beauty; yet all the years of striving for physical perfection never materialized, only reinforcing my ties to the dieting/self-hatred cycle.

Today, I don't believe I'm any different from most women in how I manage the aging process. I desire to age gracefully and am not always happy with the way my body is progressing; I have days I look in the mirror and long for the skin I had in my thirties, or even my fortes at this point. Before my 50th birthday, I decided to embrace my natural hair color despite having dyed it since I was in my early twenties. Not only was it getting harder to keep up with the growing-out process, but having placed harsh chemicals near my brain for almost thirty years, I decided my brain was more important than my vanity. Being grey at the age of fifty is not socially popular, and I found the transition uncomfortable to accept. Even though I have grown accustomed to my new look, I still have days that I wish for the youthfulness of my auburn hair. And on those days, I remind myself that "the silver-haired head is a crown of glory" (Proverbs 16:31).

Growing older is not for wimps, especially when it is not accepted as a normal part of the natural aging process

The reality is that we live in a world that values the outward appearance, but it is important for us to ask: What does God value? 1 Samuel 16:7 states that "God does not see as man sees; for man looks at the outward appearance, but God looks at the heart." As we continue reading in 1 Samuel, we see that, when God was choosing a king, He wasn't looking at the outward strength and stature of Jesse's sons. He was looking for David, the youngest son, who tended sheep. David was merely a boy who did not compare to his brothers' physical maturity, yet God saw past that. He saw the heart of a young boy that would one day be king; a boy that God would call "a man after God's own heart" (Acts 13:22).

When God sees us, He is not focused on the outer appearance or what is easily seen by man; instead His focus is on what is not easily seen: the condition of our heart. When we embark on a diet, where is our focus? Too often, every ounce of our being is engaged in the process of changing our physical appearance: what diet to choose, what to eat or not eat, how much weight to lose, dreams of a thinner body. From the time we wake to the time we climb into bed, our sole focus is on one thing and one thing only: losing weight… in other words, altering our outward appearance.

But wait! Reread 1 Samuel 16:7: "*God does not see as man sees, for man sees the outward appearance, but God sees the heart.*" God's starting line is our heart. Yet when most of us diet, changing the outer appearance becomes our beginning point, not the issues of the heart that are linked to being overweight.

Do you see the disconnect? The weight loss journey is not merely a physical issue; it includes the interconnected pieces of our spirit, soul and body. If we're going to do this diet thing differently, we must align ourselves with what God values instead of what we think has value. So as you work through the LWW, place your weight loss goal to the side and make a decision to *not* diet.

I know what you're thinking: "What? Are you kidding me? Isn't losing weight the reason I bought this book in the first place?" I know it sounds crazy not to diet or focus on weight loss when your ultimate goal is to shed pounds. It sounds like the ultimate oxymoron. So yes, the truth remains that you are overweight and you need to lose weight. But until you adjust the way you think about and relate to food and the dieting process, the kind of real, lasting change you crave will be fleeting. Your ultimate target for the next few weeks is the goal of discovery. The LWW will take you on a journey that reaches far beyond the goal of weight loss. It will be a journey to discover peace with food, the lavish love of God and a life filled with vision. And then from there, a discovery of a thinner, healthier you.

Stop dieting! Don't make your ultimate ambition weight loss. Let's do this diet thing differently.

JOURNAL

During the next four to six weeks, set aside your goal of weight loss. Put the scale away. Hide it in the attic, if needed. As God began guiding me through the healing process from my compulsive/dieting career, I got rid of the scale. Because my life had been consumed with losing weight and dieting, I needed to quit focusing on a magical number and the illusion of being model thin. If you also struggle with this unhealthy infatuation, then be willing to remove the temptation.

To begin your journey, *align* your thoughts and actions towards God's heart and what He values instead of putting all your energy and focus into weight loss. For some of you, what I am asking is HUGE! The desire to get rid of excess weight is compelling! Not making it your primary goal will be quite foreign to your typical approach to dieting. But unless you alter the starting point from weight loss to the condition of your heart, you will find yourself continually stuck in the dieting cycle.

Write a prayer expressing your desire to make 1 Samuel 16:7 the foundation of your weight loss journey. Even if you don't know what that really looks like, the key is that you remain willing and open to exploring the promises God holds for you. Below is a sample prayer:

Dear God,

Thank You for walking hand in hand with me through this wonderful weight loss transformation. I declare 1 Samuel 16:7 as the starting point, confident that I no longer have to struggle with food and dieting, but that I am free to enjoy a healthy life filled with purpose. I desire to know Your heart more than I want to lose weight or change my physical appearance. I gladly receive what You have for me, Lord: Your love, Your truth and the fulfillment of Your plans. I am ready, God!

THOUGHTS TO PONDER AS YOU JOURNAL

1. How has the media's fabricated image of beauty influenced your striving for physical change?
2. Where does dieting put your focus? How does it compare to 1 Samuel 16:7?
3. How do you feel about putting your weight loss goals on hold for the next four to six weeks? What is the benefit of doing so?

JOURNAL NOTES

~

CHAPTER 5

TAKING CONTROL

IF YOU IDENTIFY WITH THE dieter's mentality discussed in Week One, then this chapter is especially for you. We will be redesigning the "can't have" mindset by **allowing all foods!**

Yes, you heard me. All foods are permissible. I realize that all food is not created equal when it comes to nutrients; but for now, the focus rests on building a peaceful relationship with food rather than using food to lose weight.

When we deny ourselves certain foods, the compulsive eater in us will crave and obsess about the "can't haves." Then, when faced with a food that we or our current diet deem unacceptable (e.g., chocolate cake), we find ourselves engaged in a fierce mental battle...

I want.
I shouldn't.
I want.
I can't.

If we end up eating the cake, we feel guilty; and the anxiety of indulging in the "can't have" entices us to continue eating. We not only devour one piece, but two. And then we quickly proceed to shovel down the entire thing without ever allowing ourselves the pleasure of actually tasting it.

Will that one initial piece of cake make us fat? Is it the reason we're over-weight? No, it isn't. Cake is just food. It's not the problem in and of itself; therefore, it isn't what needs to be forbidden. Once we really believe that all food is acceptable, we will approach food differently. It will no longer hold the power. We will.

If certain foods are not allowed, they magnetically pull us toward them. The "can't haves" drive the desire to eat. But acceptance gives us the peace to choose what we want to eat. You *can* have that piece of cake. You will not blow your diet by doing so. You are choosing to eat a piece of food: one that may not provide nutritional benefits but is still just a piece of food in the end. We're smart enough to understand that we cannot live on nonstop junk food and expect good health, but when we give ourselves permission to enjoy all foods, we can eat with a sense of peace - without the guilt.

Again, we are in control. Not the food. Not the diet.

When you are considering eating chocolate cake or any other food that is deemed unacceptable, ask yourself: "Do I really *want* it, or am I eating it because I can't have it?" If you determine that, yes, you really do want to eat the cake, then go ahead and give yourself permission to eat it without guilt. Savor each bite. Taste the cake. Relish the flavor, but acknowledge it for what it is: a piece of cake. It does not hold the ability to make you happy, to heal your heart or to make life any better. It is simply a piece of cake you can peacefully eat and enjoy.

Once you're done, move on. If you're with friends, than enjoy the con-versation and company. If you're alone, get up from the table and start living life away from the cake. It will be there for another time. It isn't like you'll never again eat it, since it's now completely allowed. It is now a choice, not a forbidden food.

That's not to say you won't ever find yourself struggling with the old way of looking at food. I find that, even today, the former confining mindset of "shouldn't haves" creeps in. I'm free from the "can't haves," yet if I reason that I shouldn't enjoy a fattening food because it's unhealthy or I want to shed a few pounds, then I eat with a slight twinge of guilt and a yearning to eat more. I don't really take pleasure in what I'm eating because I'm not engaged in the act itself but rather in a subtle feeling that I'm doing something wrong. But when I make peace with food again, deeming all of it acceptable, I'm free to eat even what's not-so-healthy. When I'm free to choose, I'm at peace to say no. If I believe I shouldn't or can't, I'm enticed and driven to say yes.

I realize that some of you will experience a difficult time letting go of the "can't have" mentality due to the fear of being out of control, gorging on food. But the sense of rigid restriction is what drives that kind of uncontrollable behavior. There are a few foods, such as bakery cake, that I willingly choose not to eat very often because the abundance of sweet icing stirs my desire to overindulge in sugar. I still eat scrumptious cake from a bakery on special occasions, but I don't regularly keep it stocked in my food pantry.

REDESIGNING THE "CAN'T HAVES"

Even though all foods are permissible, common sense dictates that we're not going to be happy with the results if we make a habit of consuming food high in fat, calories and sugar (1 Corinthians 10:23). So how do we redesign our eating behavior to focus on foods that promote vibrant health without reinforcing the "can't have" behavior?

Our goal is to replace the least beneficial foods we eat with ones that offer greater value. Most of us won't – and shouldn't – trade every unhealthy indulgence. But we do want to begin the process of swapping out life-depleting foods with life-giving foods. The overall idea is that, instead of feeling deprived of certain choices, you control the choices that lead to change. You aren't getting rid of foods or forbidding foods, but giving yourself the power to decide which ones to replace more often than not.

Below is a list of food we typically categorize as "can't haves," followed by a list of healthier options that we can use to replace it. These two lists were adapted from a book that I recommend reading, *Greater Health God's Way-7 Steps to Inner and Outer Beauty*, by Stormie Omartian.[1] The goal is to make the "can't haves" the occasional treat and the beneficial foods the norm. The difference between this approach and all of the other, unsuccessful diets you've tried before is that you're in the driver's seat. You now have the choice to take control of the wheel and steer the direction of your health. It isn't someone else telling you what you can and cannot eat; rather, it's you designing a plan that will lead to a healthier, peaceful life.

Sitting in the driver's seat may be a scary proposition for you. It can definitely be easier to have someone else dictate what, when and how much to eat, eliminating the guesswork from the dieting process. But eventually, we grow weary of obeying the rules and we rebel. The "can't have" becomes the "I want," which eventually leads to the "I have to eat." And in the end, we reclaim control, though with an indulgent, rebellious approach. So accept that inevitable responsibility from the beginning: the control to eat what you want, when you want and how you want. The decision is not what foods you'll deny yourself, but rather what foods you'll choose to eat and, in return, how you'll design the life you desire to live. You will be amazed that, when you're in control, you'll initiate making decisions that focus on nurturing and restoring overall health and well-being.

OCCASIONAL FOODS (LIFE-DEPLETING FOODS)

1. White sugar and sugar products: jams, cakes, candies, cookies, puddings, cakes, fruits canned in sugar
2. Artificial sweeteners: aspartame, saccharine
3. White flour and white-flour products: pasta, bread
4. White rice
5. High-fat dairy products

6. Soft drinks
7. Cereals with artificial colors or sweeteners
8. Salt
9. Hydrogenated oils and saturated fats, including margarine
10. Peanut butter that is highly processed
11. Heavily processed meats: hot dogs, salami, bologna, bacon
12. Fried foods
13. "Instant" packaged foods
14. Milk chocolate
15. Canned fruit and vegetables
16. Ice cream made with chemicals
17. Coffee, tea and alcohol

REPLACEMENT FOR OCCASIONAL FOODS (LIFE-GIVING FOODS)

1. Raw honey or unrefined sugar, foods sweetened with organic cane sugar, maple syrup, honey, blackstrap molasses, fruit, fruit juice, dates, agave, stevia
2. Stevia, sugars listed above
3. Whole-grain flour: 100% whole wheat, spelt, barley, oats, millet, rye, buckwheat, whole-wheat pasta, whole-wheat or whole-grain bread, sprouted bread (you can also try spaghetti squash in place of pasta)
4. Natural brown rice, unprocessed wild rice, quinoa
5. Low-fat dairy or dairy alternatives: low-fat milk and yogurt; Greek yogurt; almond, rice or cashew milk
6. Water with a splash of juice, lemon or stevia flavored drops
7. Whole-grain cereals: Kashi, All-Bran, Uncle Sam, raw oats, whole-grain granola
8. Natural vegetable and herb seasonings, Himalayan salt, real salt, sea salt (use salt in moderation)

9. Oils that are naturally pressed and unrefined: extra virgin olive oil, coconut, canola and safflower oil
10. Natural peanut butter
11. Pure meats: look for all-meat hot dogs, bacon, etc., that are made without chemicals, sugar and nitrates
12. Baked, poached, steamed or stewed foods
13. Natural unprocessed products (e.g., buy fresh potatoes instead of instant, use real apples to make applesauce)
14. Dark chocolate, carob
15. Fresh fruits and vegetables, or frozen when fresh produce is not in season
16. Ice cream made with whole foods, such as milk, eggs and honey
17. Herb teas, organic coffee, red wine

When you review these two lists, your goal should not be to use the Replacement list 100% of the time. Certain items on the Occasional list simply won't have a replacement that works for you. That's what makes this process fun; you get to choose. If chocolate is a food you absolutely can't survive without, and dark chocolate just won't cut it, then chocolate will not have a replacement (at least most of the time). Simply realize that eating an abundance of chocolate every day will derail the path towards a healthy life. So choose to consume it wisely.

If your diet typically consists of high-fat, salty and sugary foods, than healthier options may not excite your taste buds at first. But as you transition healthier foods into your routine, your taste buds will become sensitized to the natural, unprocessed taste of food. Your cravings will lessen, and your desire for healthy choices will increase. If you want to try whole-wheat pasta but don't want to give up the "regular" kind right away, use half whole wheat and half white pasta until your taste buds adjust.

Even if you decide to stay with that half-and-half variety, your body is ultimately benefiting from an increase in nutrients. This doesn't have to be an all-or-nothing approach to your health. This isn't about perfection. This is about creating the life that you're proud to live, with your health being a blessing and not a regret.

Alignment Questions: Are you aligning yourself with the "can't have" mentality or the peace of knowing that all foods are permissible? Are you walking in the freedom to choose or giving power to the "can't haves?" Aligning yourself with the choice to replace – not forbid – food will allow you to create a healthy life of your *choosing*. You're no longer on the sidelines being told what not to eat. Now you have a front row seat in designing your life.

JOURNAL

Begin by picking one or two foods from the Occasional list and replacing them with foods from the Replacement list. Some of you will be tempted to do it all at once, taking the entire list, going on a major shopping spree and completely overhauling your kitchen cabinets. I would strongly advise against this approach. You'll end up with a huge grocery bill and a pantry full of unused food. Instead, select one or two changes to make and incorporate them into your daily routine. Ask yourself, "Can I eat this way for the rest of my life?" Making changes and dreading the taste of the healthy foods won't result in lasting change.

Give your taste buds a chance to adapt. I remember the first time I tried whole wheat bread. I didn't care for the taste until I toasted it. I now eat sprouted bread, which some people claim tastes like cardboard, but I actually enjoy it. Your taste buds can usually adjust. But if, after a valiant effort, you still find yourself gagging, then you may decide there simply is no adequate replacement for the original food.

Remember: You are free to eat it. It's permissible; you will now just have to focus on being a wise consumer of that not-so-beneficial food choice.

Have fun trying new ingredients. I remember when I first started down this road, I enjoyed discovering the nutritional benefits of new foods and attempting new recipes. This process of replacing life-depleting foods with life-giving foods is not meant to be a burden, but rather a freedom to discover and select healthy alternatives, leading to a peaceful relationship with food.

Below is an example of how you can take your daily menu and swap out healthier options from the replacement list:

Breakfast

* Toasted white bread with peanut butter and jam

Healthier Swap-out Breakfast

* 100% whole wheat bread with natural peanut butter and a drizzle of raw honey or jam sweetened with fruit juice

Lunch

* Canned soup and saltine crackers
* Turkey sandwich on white bread with mayo

Healthier Swap-out Lunch

* Homemade soup (Make a large pot of soup over the weekend so you'll have an easy grab-and-go lunch for the week. Also, skip the crackers or use a whole-grain option.)

* Whole grain bread with lettuce, mustard, turkey without nitrates, and Greek yogurt or olive-oil mayonnaise; or replace the sandwich altogether with a salad

Dinner

* Rice, chicken browned in butter, and canned veggies boiled and cooked in butter

Healthier Swap-out Dinner

* Brown rice, organic chicken sautéed in chicken broth or browned in the oven, fresh or frozen vegetables steamed or roasted in the oven with olive oil

Dessert

* A piece of chocolate cake

Healthier Swap-out Dessert

* Share the chocolate cake with a friend or two
* A piece or two of dark chocolate with a small glass of red wine
* Make a cake with healthier ingredients. Replace half of the white flour with 100% wheat, oat or spelt flour; use honey or organic cane sugar, and reduce the overall amount of sugar called for; replace all or some of the fat with applesauce; and instead of frosting, top it with whipped cream and fresh fruit.

Last but not least, here's a prayer for guidance as you redesign the "can't haves" this week:

Dear God,

Thank you that I – not the diet or food – can be in the driver's seat. Thank you that I am not denying myself but rather replacing life-depleting foods with life-giving foods, and that I have the control to design the plan that will help me achieve a healthy life. I ask that you will guide me as I decide what foods to change this week. I look forward to making changes one step at a time, which, in the end, will result in a permanent change: a peaceful, healthy relationship with food.

THOUGHTS TO PONDER AS YOU JOURNAL

1. In what ways do you relate to the "can't have" mentality?
2. How deeply is your self-perception rooted in the "can't have" mentality?
3. How do you feel when you're told that all foods are acceptable? Do you fear being out of control?
4. What is your plan for replacing life-depleting foods with life-giving foods?

JOURNAL NOTES

Week Three

CHAPTER 6

~〜୨

NECESSARY PREP TIME

BEFORE WE TACKLE IDENTIFYING THE emotional issues that keep us connected to food and dieting, it is important we have a solid understanding of who we are and the bigness of God. I want to emphasize how important this section is in preparing for Week Five, when we'll explore the question, "What am I feeding?"

You may find yourself in a hurry to simply move on and begin losing weight. You may be wondering, "Why do I have to take the time to ponder what God says about me? I already know all this stuff." But if we really understood (I mean really understood) who we are and the magnitude of the God we serve, would we continue to live in a defeated belief system? Or would we be transformed to live a life of victory?

Spend the time required this week to soak in the truth of who you are in the greatness of God! Ask God to show you "you" from His perspective. Don't rush it. Revel in it!

THE TRUTH ABOUT YOU!

What we believe about ourselves, and what we believe God says about us, significantly impacts the way we do the diet thing. Over our lifetime, we develop a set of beliefs called scripts that influence the way we think and act. These beliefs are a byproduct of our life experiences, whether positive or negative. Our future decisions and relationships will be influenced by what these scripts engrave on our hearts and souls, directly impacting the way we express and receive love.

For example, if we were raised by a loving family that instilled the values of acceptance and respect, we're more likely to develop a healthy script of "I am worthy to love and be loved," and our thoughts and actions toward ourselves and others will reflect this. Throughout life, we will gravitate towards activities and friendships that build upon our fundamental beliefs of worth and value.

The problem arises when we form the basis of our identity on negative scripts and live as though these beliefs hold validity. If we grew up being told that we are stupid and worthless, then we will have a difficult time rising above the negative belief that we are just that: insignificant and unlovable. If we don't reject these beliefs and replace them with the truth of who we are, we will act upon them, building a life based upon a perception and not an accurate picture of the truth – God's truth.

When I was growing up, my dad remarked repeatedly that, as a baby, I was so ugly that I was cute. He wasn't stating this out of cruelty, and his heart was never to hurt me. But I believed those words as my reality, and they became a part of the script that led me to believe I was never pretty or thin enough. My dad's words were not the single factor that influenced my desire for physical perfection; they were merely a part of what contributed to my self-concept. But because I accepted these words as my truth, they ultimately became my reality.

The typical script for someone who is overweight and has failed to lose it, or repeatedly loses and then regains the pounds, could sound something like this: "I blew my diet, *again*. I'm so stupid for believing I would lose the weight this time. I'll never be able to do this. I will always be fat. I'm such a failure. I hate my body. I'm so ugly and disgusting. I…hate…me."

For many of you, those thoughts are similar to what plays in your head, perhaps in smaller pieces, but loud and clear nonetheless. Ask yourself, "Is this thought pattern true?" It may be your perceived reality, but how does it compare to God's plan and purpose for your life? What determines your truth: Your perception of truth or God's truth?

Transforming the way we do this "diet thing" is recognizing the negative thought patterns that so easily filter through our mind. Our old scripts may not be easily identifiable because they're familiar and we operate in them quite comfortably. When you get up in the morning, what is the first thing you say to yourself? "Hello gorgeous/handsome" or "Oh, I feel fat today." We're used to the familiar tapes that play; we're comfortable with noticing the negative but less equipped to confess the positive. We need to recognize that our belief system, if not based on truth, is a lie.

Pause for a moment… and ask God to expose the false beliefs you so easily relate to as your truth. It's time to reject the lie and possess the truth of God's word.

Knowing what God says will help us identify the old belief scripts and replace them with what comes from the heart of God. In Ephesians 4:22-24, God says, "Put off, concerning your former conduct, the old man… and be renewed in the spirit of your mind." So let's get started living life in the truth instead of a mere perception of it.

What Does God Say About Me?

1. **I am loved by God** (1 John 3:16, Romans 5:8).

God loves you, not because of what you do for Him, but because you are His child. Think about it… The God that created every star in the heavens actually knows your name. He loves you without stipulations and with a love so deep that He was willing to send His Son to die just for you. Yet there are days we look in the mirror and have a hard time believing that we really matter or that we are good enough. To God, we count to such a degree that He demonstrated His love beyond what is easily understood. As a result, you have been redeemed and forgiven, and are a recipient of His lavish grace (Ephesians 1:7-8).

2. **I am a child of God and He is my Dad** (John 1:12, Romans 8:14-15).

Let those two truths sink in for a moment. You are a child of God – the creator of Heaven and Earth – and He is your heavenly Dad. So that makes you an heir of God (Romans 8:17) with every spiritual blessings in Christ (Ephesians 1:3). The promises of God are yours because they're a rightful inheritance of a daughter/son of God.

3. **I am fearfully and wonderfully made by God** (Psalms 139:13-14).

Not only are you His child, but you are awesomely created! He took great care to shape you so wonderfully and fearfully. Not only did He form you, but He also knows the plans for your life that are just for you (Jeremiah 29:11). His plan was not for you to wander through life questioning your purpose. Rather, the plan is there; it is yours to possess. And it is AWESOME!

Furthermore, because God loves us and He is our Dad, we can claim every promise He makes as our own. No longer do we have to base who we are on what the mirror reflects or the cultural definition of beauty, but instead our identity is defined by God's promises. Here are just a few:

- **I may approach God with boldness and confidence** (Ephesians 3:12).
- **I am more than a conqueror, and I have the victory** (Romans 8:37, 1 Corinthians 15:57).
- **I am a friend of God** (John 15:15).

- **I am chosen and appointed by God to bear His fruit** (John 15:16).
- **I am free from condemnation** (Romans 8:1).
- **I have died with Christ and died to the power of sin's rule in my life** (Romans 6:1-6).
- **I have the mind of Christ** (1 Corinthians 2:16).
- **I've been established in Christ and anointed by God** (2 Corinthians 1:21).
- **I am a new creation** (2 Corinthians 5:17).
- **I have direct access to God through the Spirit** (Ephesians 2:18).
- **God will supply all my needs** (Philippians 4:19).
- **Christ Himself is in me** (Colossians 1:27, Galatians 2:20).
- **I've been given a spirit of power, love and a sound mind** (2 Timothy 1:7).

Identify your negative belief tapes. Reject them as being your truth. Confess and believe God's word as your new truth.

I never gave much serious consideration to my dad's teasing until God revealed that his words contributed to my battle to feel loved and accepted. As soon as I recognized that, I had a choice. I could continue to accept the perceived validity of my father's words – which were spoken in jest – or I could choose to receive God's healing by rejecting my current belief and replacing it with His truth. Not only was I NOT so ugly that I was cute, but I was/am fearfully and wonderfully made by God. He formed me in my mother's womb, and He rejoices and sings over me (Psalm 139:13-14, Zephaniah 3:17).

I asked God to heal the part of me that viewed herself as a little girl who believed she was not loveable. I asked Him to speak words of love over me and to replace my father's words with His. As I asked for healing, I also proclaimed – for myself – the truth I discovered in God's Word.

Words have the power to penetrate the layers of our heart. Does that mean they hold the ability to define who we are today? Not unless we continue to give them the power to impact us by believing and acting as though they are valid.

You have a choice to make TODAY. Will you accept the past as your reality, or will you accept what God – the creator of Heaven and Earth, your heavenly Father – proclaims about you? Your circumstances may have defined the perception of truth you created and lived by for years, and it may be a comfortable place to remain; but a life dictated by the past is also a painful, weary place to stay. I could easily have chosen the old, familiar voices of un-worthiness that said I was "so ugly I was cute," but instead I decided to derive my beauty from God's glorious creation of me!

As God reveals the elements of your past that crafted your perceptions, you will also be presented with a choice. Will the familiarity of your alleged reality chain you where you are because change is uncomfortable? Or will you be brave enough to believe the untarnished truth, and strong enough to receive it as your own?

THE POWER OF THE SPOKEN WORD

> *"So is my word that goes out from my mouth: It will not return to me empty, but will accomplish what I desire and achieve the purpose for which I sent it."*
>
> *– ISAIAH 55:11*

God's word is living and powerful, sharper than a two-edged sword that pene-trates soul and spirit, and discerns the thoughts and intents of the heart (Hebrews 4:12). Speaking Scripture has the power to cut through our negative beliefs so that our identity can be transformed into the image of God. Take the time to look up each of the Scriptures listed back on pages 60-61; write them down and speak them aloud. Consider it this way… When God created the Heavens and the Earth, He spoke to bring them into existence. Today, when we are faced with insurmountable obstacles in our lives, He says we can speak to the mountains in faith and they will move. And nothing will be impossible (Matthew 17:20).

There is also the power of *life and death* in the tongue (Proverbs 18:21). When we merely *reflect* on the negative, it becomes our belief; but when we actually *speak* the negative, it sets our words into motion. The spoken word breathes life into our thoughts, releasing them into existence.

Have you ever noticed that when you're having a bad day, the more you talk and complain about it, the more defeated you become? Your day quickly spirals downward, taking with it your demeanor, behavior and actions.

In the same way, if we wake up confessing how fat we are, our words steer our thoughts and emotions. Before we know it, that single-minded negativity grows to include how we hate our hair, how overwhelmed we are at work, how our kids are driving us crazy, and how utterly wretched we feel.

I realize this may seem like an exaggeration, but take notice of the effect on your mental and emotional health the next time you speak your negative belief scripts. Instead of speaking the negative tapes of disappointment and self-hatred towards our bodies and dieting failures, let's speak the transform-ing Word of God that moves mountains! Proclaim His creative, powerful promises over your life, and be amazed at how He transforms your old nega-tive reality into His new life-changing truth.

Be aware that you may not *feel* like these Scriptures are true for you. Our emo-tions can be quite strong and real, yet contrary to God's word. When you look in the mirror and see a person who is overweight, will you profess your emotional truth that you look fat today? Or will you choose to believe what God says about you: that you are fearfully and wonderfully made? When you eat a donut at the office instead of the healthy snack you packed, will you play the failure tape that says you blew it, or will you remind yourself that you are victorious in Christ?

The old recordings will be familiar, and our emotions will want to guide our thoughts and behaviors; but we can stop these programmed scripts from playing by instead speaking God's word into and over our lives.

A word about your past: Failing at the dieting thing can encapsulate us in fear – fear we'll gain our weight back, or take a bite of food and not be able to stop. With each new attempt to lose weight, fear becomes a heavy ball and chain that weighs us down, keeping us from moving forward. Before long, our past attempts taunt us, calling us failures… telling us we're stupid to think this time will be different… that we're destined to be fat. Exhausted, our excitement wanes as our momentum breaks, and we concede to the belief that our fears are true.

But you do not have to stay locked to your past. Remember the Word of God is living and powerful, and the truth *will* set you free (John 8:32). God's Word unlocks the ball and chain that binds you to fear. However, the ability to continue walking in that renewed hope and victory depends on your willingness to fight your doubts and fears with the truth you now possess. One of the goals of the Lost Weight Workshop is to equip you to battle and break down the voice of fear. So when your past reminds you of your failures, tempting you to believe your fears are inevitable, remind it that it does not have power over you any longer. For God has not given you a spirit of fear but of love, power and a sound mind (2 Timothy 1:7).

As we increasingly become aware of who we really are, we can start our weight loss journey from a point of peace, not fear or anxiety; of victory, not defeat. If God is our heavenly Dad – who lavishly loves us, who fearfully made us, who believes in us, who we can boldly approach and who has given us the victory – then we can believe, without a shadow of a doubt, that we will succeed.

Formerly, we have strived for weight loss using a backwards approach. Our focus was on the physical while using a broken dieting system to accomplish our goal. We started out defeated. But when we first transform our spirit and soul, we can begin with the promise of victory, confident in who we are, and at peace to travel this road of weight loss and health. Any other way is putting the cart before the horse: a lot of effort with little to no return.

Alignment Questions: What am I aligning myself with, and is it producing the kind of fruit I want in my life? Am I aligning with an old, negative belief about who I am, or am I aligning myself with God's truth? Choose to renew your mind, believe the real truth and transform your identity.

JOURNAL

1. **Speak God's promises and make the following proclamation:**

"God loves ME! I am His child, a daughter/son of the King. He welcomes me into His presence and is thrilled to spend time with me. He has a plan and purpose for my life that only I can fulfill, and His plan includes me living victorious and free from the bondage to food and dieting. I am not defined by my past experiences. I choose to reject my perception of the truth and decide to believe the real truth – God's truth – of who I am."

Refer back to the identity Scriptures you wrote down; carry them with you and do not stop speaking them until your old, false belief scripts have been renewed with the knowledge of your true identity!

2. **Break off the ball and chain of your past dieting attempts.**

Speak the prayer below. Envision the chain of fear and past failures unlocking, and see yourself stepping into newfound freedom. Remember your past does not have to dictate your future. You have the victory in Christ. Don't believe anything different. When the voice of failure rises up, revisit this prayer, declaring fear's ultimate fate of defeat.

Dear God,

Thank You that my past does not have the final word on my future. You do. It is through Your Son, Jesus that I am set free (John 8:36). And in His name, I break the chains of fear that dieting has left behind. When my past reminds me of my failures, I will remind it that the victory is mine.

I recognize that I may stumble and fall as I learn to walk in the newness of doing the diet thing differently, but that does not mean failure has won. I choose to forgive myself. I will not quit. I will put my trust in You as I pick myself back up, dust myself off and claim the truth of Your Word. Fear no longer has control; instead, through Your Spirit, I walk in the power and self-discipline to overcome. Amen!

3. **Imagine God, your Heavenly Dad, writing you a love letter.**

What would it say? Write it down.

You may not be accustomed to hearing God speak words of love and affirmation over you in such a personal way, but why wouldn't He? He formed you in your mother's womb, He created you before the foundations of the earth, and He called you by name (Psalms 139:13, Ephesians 1:4, Isaiah 43:1). He is your Father and proud of it! If you've had a healthy, loving relationship with your earthly father, you may have an easier time hearing God's love letter. If your earthly dad was unable or unwilling to communicate or demonstrate love, you may find yourself challenged to write this letter. That's okay, but still give God the opportunity to express His feelings for you anyway.

If writing a love letter from God is too foreign a concept, then write from the viewpoint of what a dear and trusted friend would say about you. How does she or he see you? Write it down. Now, imagine a picture of the ideal dad. If he was to write you a love letter, what would he say? Take it one step further:

Let God be that ideal dad, and imagine what He would say about how proud He is of you and how much He loves you.

At times, I know I've found it difficult to imagine God speaking to me in such an intimate manner. So I begin the process by remembering specific words my dad spoke to me in the latter years of his life.

My parents retired in Pennsylvania in close proximity to me and my family, and I would frequently stop by to visit them. On numerous occasions, my dad made an effort to remind me that he was so proud of the woman I had become. His proclamation of love was not based on my performance or my accomplishments, but based on the fact that I was simply his daughter.

That's how it's supposed to be; how it was designed to be. Yet how many times do we equate God's affection for us with our performance or accomplishments rather than just the fact that we're His children?

My letter from God might start out something like this: "To my sweet daughter, I just want you to know how proud I am of you. I am proud to be your Dad and to call you my daughter..."

Take time to listen to what God really has to say about you. You will be amazed at the depth of His love and how precious you are to Him. Regularly reread your letter, especially on days when discouragement creeps in or when the old scripts are rising up to defeat you.

THOUGHTS TO PONDER AS YOU JOURNAL

1. What beliefs or experiences have influenced the way you think about yourself?
2. How do these beliefs manifest in the outworking of your life?
3. In what ways do you identify with the typical dieter's script?

4. What does your script in particular sound like?

5. When you read that you are loved by God, that you're His child and are fearfully made by Him, what does that mean to you?

6. Name three things that God says about you, and replace three negative thoughts you have of yourself.

7. Write down and memorize three Scriptures to confess out loud when you find yourself operating in your old, defeated thought pattern.

RECOMMENDED READING FOR WEEK THREE

For the ladies: *Captivating: Unveiling the Mystery of a Woman's Soul* by John and Stasi Eldredge.

For the men: *Wild at Heart: Discovering the Secret of a Man's Soul* by John Eldredge.

JOURNAL NOTES

Week Four

CHAPTER 7

The Wrong Key

Food plays a vital role in our lives: to provide essential nutrients that nourish our physical body. These nutrients promote good health and are vital to our existence, but food positively cannot – in any way, shape or form – heal the brokenness of our lives; it is fundamentally impossible. It simply lacks the capacity to fill this void. Yet for many of us, we continue to use food to meet our emotional needs, a role that is absolutely beyond the scope of its ability to fulfill.

Imagine yourself pouring out your heart about a difficult situation in your life to one of your dearest friends. Maybe you're stressed at work or school, had an argument with your spouse or are worried about one of your kids. You completely trust this friend to listen empathetically and to offer sound advice. After you've finished sharing your concerns, your friend gives you the following anointed words of wisdom: "Go brush and floss your teeth." Your friend continues to reassure you that not only will you feel better, but this simple act of brushing and flossing will heal your emotional pain and relieve your stress. At this point, you're probably thinking that your friend has completely lost it, and you're asking "What in the world does brushing and flossing my teeth have to do with making my heart feel better?"

Exactly!

The act of taking care of our teeth plays an essential role in dental hygiene, a function that is physical, but not emotional or spiritual. To think otherwise would be absurd. Isn't it just as ridiculous that we choose to use food – which also has a purely physical function – to heal the emotional pain we experience in life? It's just as silly as reaching for dental floss. I hope we can laugh together at this example, because at some point, we're all guilty of this emotional forgery. But where does this leave us?

Trying to fill an emotional void with something that emphatically will not work is like trying to open a locked door with the wrong key. No matter how many times we try the key, it won't open the door, and we find ourselves frustrated and shut out from where we want to be.

When we use food as the solution to our feelings, we're using the *wrong* key. Food is not the ingredient that can make sadness disappear, bring true joy, relieve stress or restore loss. What it will do is make us weary of repeatedly trying to unlock the issues of the heart with no real hope of success.

A popular definition of insanity is doing the same thing over and over again, and expecting different results. And how many of us feel like we're going crazy trying to diet because we continue to feed our heart while expecting a different end result? The key we're using to meet our emotional needs will never bring about the change we so desperately desire.

All keys begin with a basic form and are molded and shaped by a craftsman. Each one is ground perfectly to fit the opening of its intended lock; and so it is with the one that opens our hearts. Each one of us has our own unique needs; and God, the master craftsman, knows exactly how to create the precisely shaped key to unlock our deepest desires.

That sounds beautiful, I know. And it is. But also consider this: When a key is put in the metal grinder, it makes an uncomfortable sound and bits of itself are removed to make it unique. As we go through the process of letting

God mold our means of escape – our means to freedom – we may feel uncomfortable with the shaping process. Remember though: In the beginning of this book, we asked God to plow up the fallow ground of our hearts. We know that in order for the true beauty of our hearts to shine forth, the messy parts must undergo the difficult shaving and reshaping process.

God's love is so perfect for bringing healing to our hearts. He created us with great skill and precision. Who better to meet our innermost longings? No one else knows exactly what we need at each precise moment in time. He is the one that heals our brokenness and binds up our wounds (Psalm 147:3). He has given us the key: His love. Will we accept it and allow Him to uniquely shape it for us?

Finally, a Good Reason to Celebrate Fat!

"Because Your love is better than life, my lips will glorify You. I will praise You as long as I live, and in Your name I will lift up my hands. My soul will be satisfied as with the richest of foods; with singing lips my mouth will praise You."

– Psalms 63:3-5

In the NKJV, that passage reads, "My soul shall be satisfied with fat and abundance."

As you read the above cited Scripture, how comforting to know that God's love will satisfy your soul as if you were feasting on the richest foods, feeling fat and abundantly full!

Imagine your favorite Thanksgiving meal: the bounty of your treasured family foods, the comfort of loved ones, the satisfaction of being truly blessed with abundance. That feeling is a small comparison to the fulfillment of

God's love. Instead of using food to satisfy the longing of our hearts and plug the void, God promises that His love – which is better than life – will not only satisfy our hearts, but fill it with fat and abundance. I love how God doesn't give us just enough of His love, but He gives until we are overflowing with its fullness (Ephesians 3:19).

Just as the dietary fat we consume in our food helps to generate feelings of satiation and satisfaction, God's love satisfies the hunger of our heart. The reason low-fat diets fail is because, without fat, we continue to feel unfulfilled and long for more to eat. So fat is essential, not only in the natural, but especially if it's God's fat. God's love *will* satisfy our soul; His love *will* comfort, heal and satiate our innermost being.

Refer back to the second half of Psalms 63:3-5. It speaks of praise and thanksgiving, which are essential parts of experiencing God's overflowing love: "I will praise you as long as I live… with singing lips my mouth will praise you."

I know when life gets tough, an attitude of thanksgiving is the last thing we *feel* like doing, and it can be challenging for praise to roll off our lips. It is easier to speak the reality of what we are feeling – the pain, sadness or disappointment – rather than God's truth. If we're to experience God's abundant, ever-present love that is better than life, we need to decide to praise God for who He is and who we are in Him.

I believe that David, when he wrote the Psalms, provided a perfect example. David was always honest with God about his circumstances and how he felt in the midst of his turmoil. He didn't hold back; he would pour out his heart honestly and boldly before God. Take Psalm 57:4, for example, where he essentially cried out, "Lord, I'm in the midst of lions and ravenous beasts!" But no matter how bad his circumstances were (facing lions – whether real or metaphorical – counts for a pretty bad day, in my opinion), he always chose to praise and confess the goodness of God. "I will praise you, O Lord" he wrote, "… for great is your love, reaching to the heavens; your faithfulness reaching to the skies" (Psalm 57: 9-10 NIV).

He knew the goodness of God and made a conscious decision to praise Him even in the toughest of situations. As you experience hardships, it is tempting to wallow in the pain. Instead, *honestly* acknowledge the pain and take it a step further to proclaim – with a heart of praise and thanksgiving – who God *is* in your circumstances. This simple, but not always easy, action will open your heart to the outpouring of God's love. Take time to read the Psalms and learn from David, a man after God's own heart.

JOURNAL

As you work through this next section – answering the question of "What am I feeding?" – ask God to reveal instances where you substituted food for His love. Where you've used food as the key to your stress, hurt, fear or pain, grant this position of honor to God, allowing Him to heal your heart. Use your journal to write down what God reveals to you.

Make this prayer your declaration:

Dear God,

Wow! How abundant is Your love for me! Thank You for Your love that is better than life. Forgive me for using food to bring healing and wholeness to my circumstances. I choose to no longer use food to meet my emotional needs, and will not put it in a role that is impossible for it to fulfill. I ask You to fill my heart so that I will be satisfied in a way I have never known. Your love will be the key that unlocks and heals my heart. Thank You for filling me with your fat. Finally, a good reason to be fat! Amen!

Alignment Questions: What am I aligning myself with, and is it producing the kind of fruit I want in my life? Am I aligning myself with using food to meet my emotional needs, or am I aligning myself with God's love as the key to my heart?

THOUGHTS TO PONDER AS YOU JOURNAL

1. When do you find yourself eating to meet your emotional needs instead of your physical ones?
2. How do you use food as the key to quiet the cry of your heart?
3. Using food to fill the pain or emptiness is emotional forgery. What does that mean to you?
4. Psalm 63:5 says that God's love is better than life and will satisfy us with fat and abundance. What would it feel like to experience a love like that in your life?
5. In what areas do you need God's love to satisfy you with fat and abundance?
6. Take notice of your thoughts and spoken words. Do you have a David's heart of praise, or do you find yourself complaining or dwelling in the circumstances of your heart?

JOURNAL NOTES

~?

CHAPTER 8

DISCOVERING A BIGGER GOD!

LET'S TAKE A DEEPER LOOK into the concept of alignment and how it can impact our perception of God. If you think God can't handle the circumstances of your life – that your physical, emotional and spiritual burdens weigh too much – then get ready to think again.

Several years ago, there was a popular book written that contended we can create the life we desire by using three simple steps: Ask, believe and receive. This line of reasoning – which is still around today – says that, if we make a command to the universe, letting it know what we want and believing we've already received our request, the universe will give a positive answer.[1]

Yet what is the universe? *Webster's Dictionary* defines it as "the entire celestial cosmos; all of space and everything in it, including stars, planets, galaxies, etc.; the whole body of things and phenomena observed or assumed."[2] In that case, the theory above sounds pretty cool. But I have one better, and it's based on a relationship, not a philosophy. God, your *heavenly Dad*, is the creator of the universe. Take a moment for that to sink in. God, the creator of Heaven and Earth and the entire celestial cosmos, just happens to also be your Father!

Why would we align ourselves with the universe when we personally know its *creator*?

The satellites we have today are providing new insight into the grandeur of what's beyond our tiny planet. Scientists are discovering how vast it actually is and how much is yet to be discovered. Our human minds have a hard time grasping concepts that do not fit neatly into the limited realm of what we can see or understand.

When you consider God, how big is your view? Do you equate Him with the simple songs you sang as a child, believing His love to be meek and mild? Do you see His power and majesty as something that fits neatly and finitely in the understanding of your mind?

We sometimes tend to restrict who He is based on our narrow view or lack of understanding, but God and His love are infinite, everlasting and never changing. God and His love are BIG! They are wider, longer, higher and deeper than we can truly comprehend. Because of His great love, we're able to accomplish infinitely more than we might ask or think. Infinitely more! (Ephesians 3:17-21 NLT).

If your view of God is based on what you learned as a young child, or if He fits in the narrow scope of what you have imagined, it's time to discover the bigness of God. He is everything you need to be victorious on the weight loss journey. No matter what you face, He has the answer.

Below are just a few Scriptures that describe who He is. I encourage you to write them down, meditate on them and, when you feel defeated, declare the bigness of God into your circumstances. Work on spending less time praying about your circumstances and more time praying *who God is* **into** your circumstances. As you delve into the Word of God, you will continue to discover a greater depth of understanding of His greatness. I also encourage you to do a study of the names of God, which will further enrich your understanding of who He is.

Scriptures for Discovering a Bigger View of God

- God is my refuge and strength (Psalm 46:1, Psalm 28:7, Habakkuk 3:19).
- God is my fortress (Psalm 18:2).
- God is my strong tower (Psalm 61:3, Proverbs 18:10).
- God is my deliverer (Psalm 34:19, Psalm 18:2, 2 Samuel 22:2, Psalm 140:7).
- God is my healer (Exodus 15:26, Psalm 34:18, Psalm 30:2, 1 Peter 2:24).
- God goes before me and is my rear guard (Isaiah 58:8, 52:12).
- God is my comforter (John 14:26, Psalm 147:3).
- God is my provider (Philippians 4:19, Psalms 34:10-12).
- God is my rescuer (2 Samuel 22:3).
- God is my savior (Psalm 79:9, Psalm 25:5, Psalm 38:22, 1 Timothy 4:10, Isaiah 45:21).

So… Who is your God? If your belief in Him is bound by limitations or you've allowed it to diminish over time, remind yourself of who God really is: a God of love and a whole lot more!

You may experience difficulty believing that you can conquer the weight loss battle because you've aligned yourself with the dieting system for so long and with such limited success. But if we truly align ourselves with God's heart and the bigness of His love, He guarantees that we can accomplish infinitely more than we might ask or believe. If that doesn't sound like success, I don't know what does.

So yes, let's ask, believe and receive. But instead of asking a celestial cosmos, let's ask, believe and receive from the God who created it all, who promises us a love that is far better than life, and who fills us with abundance (Psalms 63:3-5).

Alignment Questions: Have you aligned yourself with a small-god belief, or are you aligning yourself under the truth of the magnitude of God? Do you accept your circumstances as "the way it is," or do you believe "who God is" and pray the bigness of God into your circumstances?

JOURNAL

Look up the above-mentioned Scriptures. Write them down and meditate on them. Begin to pray and speak the bigness of God over your life and circumstances. If God is our deliverer, rescuer and strength, and we believe we have victory in Him, then why do we accept anything less?

THOUGHTS TO PONDER AS YOU JOURNAL

1. When you think of God in relationship to the problems in your life, how big or small is your view of God?
2. Write down three Scriptures that help to expand your image of God.
3. Where in your life do you need to spend less time praying about your circumstances and more time praying God *into* your circumstances?
4. Watch the YouTube video *Indescribable* by Louie Giglio. (Don't skip this video. It will blow your mind!) Describe the bigness of God in your own words.

JOURNAL NOTES

Week Five

CHAPTER 9

~✎

"WHAT AM I FEEDING?"

EVEN WHEN WE LOGICALLY REALIZE that cookies and chips can never heal our emotions, we still may find ourselves using food to medicate and numb our hearts. For me, sugar was my drug of choice. When others turned to pills or alcohol to suppress the pain, I resorted to food. If you use food to medicate your feelings, you will want to start seeking the reason by asking the question, "What am I feeding?"

Asking the question will take courage, but uncovering the motivation for this behavior is essential to breaking the dieting cycle. The overuse of food will simply mask or compress the pain, never completely heal it. It can numb our emotional cravings for a time at least, but the wound still exists. Food is just a temporary fix to our hearts' cry, but God is the one who can completely restore the cracks and brokenness in our lives. If you're willing to ask God the difficult questions and accept the answers He lovingly provides, then you'll discover the precise key that fits the deepest parts of your heart.

As you ask the question, "What am I feeding?" write down when you witness a reliance on food as a substitute key. What is the voice within your heart that cries out but is suppressed with food? What are you afraid of feeling or discovering? Where does the fear come from that keeps you tied to your layers of fat?

Do you drown your loneliness with pizza when you're home on a Friday night and your friends are out on dates? Do you reach for the carton of ice cream after an argument with your husband? Do you demolish a plate of nachos because your boss rejected your creative ideas? Ask yourself: Are you eating because you're feeling alone or upset, or is there a deeper emotional void you're feeding?

In the earlier years of my marriage, I avoided conflict like the plague. I was a peacekeeper at all costs. Growing up, conflict in my family was negative and something to be avoided. My husband on the other hand, being from New Jersey, had conflict imprinted on his DNA. (No offense to those of you who share that state.) When John and I disagreed, I didn't know how to handle the emotions that arose. Instead of speaking up to discuss the issues, thereby risking rejection, I responded by manipulating what was in my ability to control. Food was the one thing I could control; my husband's response was not.

At that point in my life, I was no longer a compulsive eater, but eating cookies – even just an extra handful or two to numb my heart – was still giving food the authority to do something it was incapable of doing: healing my heart, something only God can truly do.

Over the years, God has revealed that the deeper issue was not the disagreement with my husband, but the fear of rejection and the attempt to control negative circumstances. As God healed my heart, He gave me the courage to make different choices. Even though it wasn't always easy, I knew I had to work through the conflict rather than stuffing my feelings down with food.

There was another period in my life where I once again resorted to using food to mask my feelings. I had adopted a vegetarian lifestyle and found it quite intriguing to incorporate unique, healthy foods into my diet. But as I experienced a rough patch in life, I *unknowingly* sought to control what was in my realm of influence. I felt powerless in my overarching circumstances and for a season, instead of overcompensating with food, I took it to the extreme by eating a strict vegan diet. The problem was not the vegan lifestyle, but that I was doing it in an unhealthy way.

The more significant part of the problem involved my reasoning; I believed that if I could follow what I (and some fellow Christian health ministries) considered to be the healthiest and godliest approach to eating, than I would somehow be more acceptable to God. At the core of my heart was a longing to be loved and accepted, which I tried to fulfill by striving for physical perfection. I had moved from the teen years of seeking approval by the world's standards of thinness, to a young woman striving for God's acceptance by attaining the purist way of eating.

I was unaware of my heart's hidden agenda. The heart is tricky that way. It was only through giving God permission to dig up the unknown parts of my heart that His love revealed what was buried deep within.

Today, God has healed the places of my heart that longed for love and acceptance. I accept that God loves me, not through personal efforts but in being and resting in Him. I'm positive that God will reveal more areas of my life that need His healing touch of love; but I'm happy to know that, today, I am completely and radically loved and adored by the most awesome God who just happens to be my heavenly Dad. And so are you! It just doesn't get any better than that!

The reason I fed my heart the wrong ingredients wasn't because of an argument or life's circumstances, but rather due to the fear of rejection, the longing for love and acceptance, and my effort to control what I could. You may overeat because you're stressed, sad, bored or angry; and that may be all there is to it. But be willing to ask God, "Is there more? Is the reason I'm eating too much because I'm feeding the deeper issue of my heart?"

As I write this book, I have a nagging twenty pounds that I've lost on several occasions; yet I find they keep reappearing. I've been attributing this to common issues, such as lack of time to exercise and poor planning. That's somewhat true, but God revealed a deeper issue at hand. While writing the "What Am I Feeding" section, God reminded me that when I initially gained the weight, a painful life event had occurred; and each time this difficult situation returns, I gain the weight back.

The deeper problem is not a lack of discipline in regards to my eating. Rather, it's a particular life event that triggers my battle with the inability to control painful circumstances and the fear of rejection. Even though I possess no guarantee that this event won't occur again, I know I do not have to remain in this cycle.

Let me be clear: Even though God miraculously set me free from the bondage to food and dieting in my twenties, I still have a choice today as to whether I use food to numb my heart. The difference is that now, food no longer controls me. I'm not addicted to food and dieting, and my self-esteem is no longer wrapped around being thin.

But when I do find myself overeating, I have to be willing to ask the question of "What am I feeding?" And I need to be astute enough to listen to the answer. Then God can reveal the issues of my heart (the unrest, anxiety, stress, etc.) that drive the desire to eat in an attempt to bury my feelings deep inside.

Once I recognize the real issue at hand, I'm presented with a choice: to continue eating… or to take what's eating at me to God, knowing that, when I feel out of control, He is in control. When I feel rejected, I am accepted by Him. His love is the key to my heart, not food. To permanently lose these twenty pounds, I am changing my response from food to a reliance on God to protect and cover me through the painful circumstances of life.

JOURNAL

As you explore the answers to why you eat, your emotional pain will raise its ugly head and a natural response will be to stuff food in your mouth, creating another safe, protective layer to quiet the pain. It's time to let the pain rise up instead of repressing it. It's time to let it surface, to reveal the festering wound and to allow God the opportunity to do what He loves to do… to heal the brokenhearted, to restore what the locusts have eaten, and to breathe new life into what we deem as dead (Psalm 147:3, Joel 2:25). If you continue to stuff your wounds with food, you'll prevent those areas that need care from surfacing. Be brave enough to stop stuffing. Be brave enough to start healing.

Ask the question, "What am I feeding?" and write down your answer. What surrounds your desire to eat? Journal freely; don't edit your responses. God may uncover specific words or memories that created an emotional void.

Was there a significant life event or trigger that happened around the time you started gaining weight? Are you building protective layers to hide from the pain of a hurtful relationship, like an overbearing mom or an absent father? Have you experienced significant loss or physical or emotional abuse?

Write down any distinct memory, action or words that are exposed. Explore what you discover. I'm amazed at the power of words to leave a lasting imprint on our hearts. A woman attending one of my health classes shared a story about facing ridicule for being fat when she was a young girl. Even though she was in her mid-forties, her eyes were filled with tears of pain as if the ordeal happened yesterday.

AREAS TO EXPLORE IN RELATION TO ANSWERING THE QUESTION OF "WHAT AM I FEEDING?"

* Significant life events
* Relationships
* Spoken Words
* Hurtful actions

The response that leads you to the kitchen when faced with an emotional issue is too often second nature. You'll need to become aware of what's motivating you to eat. Is it actual hunger? Is it an emotional response? Once you're able to recognize that your actions are tied to emotions, you can begin addressing these difficult feelings. At this point, you'll be at a crossroads of whether to remain rooted in the emotional food cycle or to rest in the security of God's love, trusting Him to reveal the deeper issue of your heart.

Choose to speak and believe God's truth over your life and into your circumstances. Ask Him to give you a specific promise to stand firm on when you find yourself wanting to fall back to previous unhealthy habits. This process may be difficult and uncomfortable, but figuring out why you use food as the key to your pain is worth the effort. It will open the depths of your heart to a new joy and freedom. Then you will truly comprehend that only one key was ever needed: God's love.

THOUGHTS TO PONDER AS YOU JOURNAL

1. Can you identity a specific time when your weight began to increase?
2. Was there a significant life event or trigger that happened around this time?
3. Are your protective layers in place to hide the pain from hurtful relationships?

4. Have you experienced significant loss, or physical or emotional abuse?
5. What areas of your life do you use food to numb the pain of your heart?
6. Is food a way for you to control your circumstances? Or is it one aspect of your life that you use to feel in control?
7. What does eating because you're hungry feel like? What does eating because you're emotional feel like?

JOURNAL NOTES

~⁀

CHAPTER 10

FORGIVENESS IS PART OF THE KEY

AS YOU WORK THROUGH THE journal section of Chapter Nine, you may uncover how other people's words or actions have left a residue of hurt or a deep-seated pain within your heart. You will be faced with the sometimes difficult yet necessary step of forgiveness. Forgiving someone who hurt you is not easy, especially if the harm was intentional, but the act of forgiveness is not considered optional if you hope to move beyond the pain of the offense.

The reason I choose to make forgiveness a fundamental principle of my faith is twofold. First, God commands us to forgive (Matthew 6:14, Colossians 3:13). Second, I don't want anything to distance me from my relationship with God. I want my heart to be right in His eyes.

I also know that holding grudges causes no pain to the other person; it only hurts me. It keeps me bound in my hurt and brokenness, unable to receive healing to that part of my heart. Over time, these feelings turn to bitterness, a heart condition that spews out and defiles many (Acts 8:23, Hebrews12:15). Facial expressions, attitudes and actions reveal the heart of a bitter person. Have you ever noticed how individuals who cling to a heart filled with anger and pain age with wrinkles of bitterness?

I sure don't want to end up as a bitter, old, wrinkled woman. More importantly, I don't want to be emotionally locked up, unable to receive the love of my heavenly Father. I desire to be right with God more than I desire to be right.

If you've been hurt, realize you will need to forgive. The act of forgiveness is not based on a feeling or an emotion, but it occurs when we step out in faith with an obedient heart. Forgiveness may not always be easy, but a prayer of forgiveness is simple:

"God, by faith and out of obedience to You, I choose to forgive (insert name)_____ for (insert action) _____. I ask You to heal my heart, my mind and my emotions; and bring me to a place where my emotional healing matches my obedience to forgive."

I've been amazed at how God heals my emotions so that I don't continue to feel the pain of the offense done to me. Sometimes the healing is immediate, but often it requires more time because of the depth of the wound. Yet when we take that first step of obedience to forgive, God gently embraces our heart, healing its deepest cry.

Don't miss out on what God has for you because you think someone is undeserving of forgiveness. Remember: "For all have sinned and fall short of the glory of God" (Romans 3:23). The act of forgiveness is less about the other person, and more about your personal healing and freedom.

*J*OURNAL

Ask God to reveal any person or situation that has hurt or offended you. Step out in faith to speak a simple prayer of forgiveness, similar to the one above. Ask God to heal the parts of your heart and mind that have been impacted. Let His healing love break down the walls and restore the brokenness of your heart. Be patient with yourself if you still experience negative feelings tied to the offense. Keep releasing them back to God, and know that your emotional healing will come in alignment with your step of obedience. Forgiveness does not mean we forget; but with forgiveness, the emotional sting of the offense is healed, freeing us from lingering pain and emotional damage.

Alignment Questions: What am I aligning myself with, and is it producing the kind of fruit I want in my life? Am I aligning myself with hurt from my past, either in words spoken or actions against me? Am I aligning myself with bitterness, or am I choosing to forgive those who offended me?

THOUGHTS TO PONDER AS YOU JOURNAL

1. What does forgiveness mean to you?
2. Do you see forgiveness as a choice or a commandment?
3. What keeps you from choosing to forgive those who hurt you?
4. How can forgiveness free you to experience more of what God has for you?

JOURNAL NOTES

_____

_____

_____

_____

_____

_____

_____

_____

_____

_____

_____

_____

_____

_____

_____

_____

_____

_____

_____

_____

_____

_____

_____

_____

_____

_____

~~~

CHAPTER 11

Checking Your Alignment

As we discussed earlier, we are created as a complex being with the interconnected pieces of spirit, soul and body. Have you ever considered in what order these three parts of our being should be aligned?

When we diet, we have a tendency to make our body front and center. Our focal point is the physical, from the moment we wake until we crawl into bed. What we look like, whether we lost weight, what food we eat or avoid, how we feel in our clothes, and whether our pants fit loose or snug... It's all about the physical.

If that's the case, we find ourselves focused less on what matters to God, which is our heart (1 Samuel 16). We lose sight of the bigger picture, and we develop tunnel vision, focused on one thing and one thing only: losing weight. At this point, we are certainly out of alignment.

Second in line is our soul (emotions, mind and will). How much time do we spend emotionally focused on the process of losing weight? Again, from the instant we rise to the moment we fall asleep, our thoughts are consumed with dieting. We jump on the scale, and whether the number reflects a loss or gain determines our degree of mental and emotional investment for the day.

From there, we spend time obsessing over our food choices, whether they were good or bad, and whether we performed well. We may feel happy because we made healthy choices and can now envision a thin body. But if we performed poorly, we spend a huge chunk of mental and emotional energy in the unhealthy guilt and condemnation cycle. We allow our emotions and our thoughts to determine what choices we make and whether we'll psychologically beat ourselves up through the process.

Are the body and soul to be the front runners of our lives? Are we led by our emotions and the physical, or by our spirit? Does the body and soul determine our choices, our behavior and our beliefs? Or does our spirit lead the way while guided by the Spirit of God?

Our spirit, when aligned with God's, is where true transformation takes place. When placed in the position to lead, our spirit will speak truth when our emotions tell us differently. It will renew our thought life from one of defeat to victory, and will take our focus off the temporary goal of weight loss to ones of eternal value.

As you're on this journey, it's easy to get out of alignment. It's normal to put the physical first because our desire is to change our appearance. It's familiar to make this an emotional experience because our hearts are deeply invested in the process, not to mention how easy it is to become mentally preoccupied during the dieting journey. But if we allow ourselves to be led by these parts of our being instead of the spirit, we'll continue to remain trapped in the dieting cycle.

When I find that I'm out of alignment, I speak a simple prayer where I call my spirit to attention. I command my soul and body to get in line and resume their proper places. I bless my spirit and ask it to be sensitive to, and be led by, the Holy Spirit.

I have found this prayer to be helpful in other areas of my life as well. When I walked through an intense, emotionally invested time in my marriage, it was natural to walk in the pain and make decisions based on my feelings. Even though I allowed myself the freedom to feel and acknowledge those emotions, I refrained from allowing them to dictate my thoughts or decisions. I chose to have my spirit rise up so that I could discern the truth based on God's word – not based on a heart overflowing with emotions.

Emotions are real, but they don't necessarily line up with God's word. The emotionally invested dieter will continue to live defeated, allowing feelings to dictate their health, and guide their choices of whether to eat life-giving food or drown life's sorrows with chocolate. If we allow our soul to rule, we'll continue riding the crazy, merry-go-round of dieting.

JOURNAL

If you have allowed your thoughts, emotions or body to lead the weight loss journey, it's time to realign yourself. Allow your spirit to lead and the rest to follow.

A simple prayer of alignment: *Spirit, rise up and come to the forefront. I align you before my soul and body. Take your proper place and be sensitive to the Holy Spirit, ready to receive God's best.*

To bless your spirit daily, I recommend a powerful little book called, *Daily Spirit Blessings* by Arthur Burk and Sylvia Gunter. I have found the prayers offered in this book to be instrumental in keeping my spirit aligned and uplifted, and I believe you will as well.

THOUGHTS TO PONDER AS YOU JOURNAL

1. When you've dieted in the past, what part of you leads: mind, emotions, body or spirit? How so?
2. What would it look like for you to approach weight loss with your spirit leading the way?

JOURNAL NOTES

_____

_____

_____

_____

_____

_____

_____

_____

_____

_____

_____

_____

_____

_____

_____

_____

_____

_____

_____

_____

_____

_____

_____

_____

_____

_____

_____

Week Six

~

CHAPTER 12

PREPARING YOUR HEALTH ROOM

As WE CONTINUE ON THIS journey of discovering how to do the "diet thing" differently, we will need the wisdom and knowledge to complete it. If I asked you what you know about dieting, what foods are considered healthy, which carbs are good or bad, how many servings of fruits and vegetables should be consumed daily, what is good fat versus bad fat... you would probably be able to write an entire book with your collection of data. Knowledge, we have. Books, magazines and the media throw a continual bombardment of nutrition and health facts, figures and opinions at us. We don't need more information regarding how to lose weight and eat healthy, but we do need the type of knowledge that will transform our old way of doing things.

God commands us to get wisdom and understanding (Proverbs 4:5). He says that, "Through wisdom a house is built, and by understanding it is established; by knowledge the rooms are filled with all precious and pleasant riches" (Proverbs 24:3-4). God used these three principles for creation as well. "By wisdom He founded the Earth; by understanding He established the Heavens; by His knowledge the depths were broken up, and the clouds drop down the dew" (Proverbs 3:19-20). So I think we can conclude that they're important to ponder.

Proverbs tells us that when God builds a house, He uses knowledge to fill the rooms with all precious and pleasant riches; or as the NIV translation states..."with rare and beautiful treasures" (24:3-4). Now use yourself as an analogy for the house, with your health representing a room inside. Based on the knowledge you have, what does this room look like? Take stock of your current health, and use the symbolism of furniture and décor to describe it. Does your health represent a room filled with beauty, peace, comfort and energy? Or does it look tired, neglected, sickly and dingy? Is it a place you would enjoy spending time in?

As I age, I desire my health to be a room filled with brightness and vitality. I don't want to settle for old, deteriorating décor because of misuse or neglect from adhering to a pattern of fruitless thinking. And I don't want you to settle either.

So the question is, how do we take the earthly knowledge we have about eating healthy and infuse it with God's precious riches of knowledge? God speaks about being transformed by the renewing of our mind; of putting off the old man (the old way we think about dieting and weight loss) to be renewed in the spirit of our mind and put on the new man (a new way of thinking about ourselves and weight loss). Ephesians 4:22-24 (NIV) says we are to be made new in the *"attitude"* of our minds. As you read these next sections, let God renew your thoughts and attitudes about the precious gifts of knowledge He has given you, so that your health room will be filled with rare and beautiful treasures.

Gift or Heavy Backpack?

Do you ever feel like the goal of weight loss is a tedious task? Has doing all the "right things" for your health become a burdensome backpack you carry rather than a lifestyle that flows from within? Each day, you fill your backpack with all the right stuff: eating the appropriate amount of fruits and veggies, drinking eight glasses of water, consuming only whole grain, choosing lean protein and exercising at least three times per week.

After you've filled your pack with all the "right things," you put it on and begin your day. Before long, you feel the burden of trying to manage your daily health to-dos. Some days, you find yourself at the end, only to realize that your backpack is still full. Full of the fruits and veggies you didn't have time to eat, the water that sits untouched, and the healthy lunch you swapped out for a fast-food hamburger. And of course, you're too exhausted to touch the exercise at the bottom of the pack. As you pass out on the bed, you hope that tomorrow will be different. That, just maybe, you'll manage to unpack your heavy backpack and complete your health to-do list.

I don't believe God ever intended for our health to be a burden. His ways are not heavy and burdensome. For He says, "Take My yoke upon you and learn from Me, for I am gentle and lowly in heart, and you will find rest for your souls. For My yoke is easy and My burden is light" (Matthew 11:29-30).

Can our health be a part of our life that flows out of a greater purpose rather than something we put on and strive to accomplish throughout our day? Can our health be a byproduct of who we are instead of a to-do list to accomplish? I believe it can, but we will need to change the game plan and purpose for losing weight.

REDIRECTING YOUR MOTIVATION

When we've failed at losing weight in the past, what do we ultimately do? We pick a new diet to follow. This alters the game plan, but the goal and motivation remain the same: to lose weight.

But has this strategy of keeping weight loss (which is a shortsighted goal) as the motivation and *only* changing the diet plan produced lasting success?

If you're reading this book, I assume your answer is "not much, if any." So if weight loss is a temporary goal that has failed to yield permanent results, maybe we should be less concerned with picking a new diet, and instead redirect our motivation to an objective with a greater purpose and lasting impact.

When we get to Heaven, God won't be focused on our physical exterior. We've already looked at 1 Samuel 16, which shows how He doesn't look at the outward appearance but sees the heart. God isn't going to keep a record of the weight we lost, or praise us because we managed to look younger than our actual age. He will, however, be pleased that we were good stewards with the bodies He provided, and that we loved ourselves enough to nourish our physical health.

With this demonstration of love, we'll possess the energy, and mental and spiritual clarity to accomplish the plans and purpose God holds for us. I can only imagine the sadness God feels over lives that were cut short due to the complications of obesity. "He knows the plans He has for us, plans to prosper us and not to harm us" (Jeremiah 29:11, NIV). He knows the destiny He has planned for us; and how sad to see a life unfulfilled due to preventable sickness and disease.

What kind of life do you envision living? When you think of your weight loss goals, what do you visualize? Do you see yourself looking fashionable in a pair of skinny jeans or bathing suit, or in a suit and tie for a special occasion? These are short-term goals. Once reached, they rarely provide lasting results.

The vision for our lives reaches far beyond that of just weight loss. We have a powerful purpose. If we could just grab hold of the awesomeness of God's plans, our motivation for health would reach far beyond looking good in our clothes and carrying a heavy backpack of to-dos… and be more about creating a life filled with hopes and dreams for the future. To do the diet thing differently, we will need to expand our vision from weight loss to one of eternal value with the potential to impact, not only our lives, but generations to come.

God is clear that a people without vision will perish (Proverbs 29:18 KJV). If we lack vision, we'll lack the direction to accomplish anything beyond the ordinary in our lives. Mark Batterson, in his book *The Circle Maker*, compares the brain to a goal-seeking organism. He asserts that, "Setting a goal creates structural tension in your brain, which will seek to close the gap between where you are and where you want to be, who you are and who you want to become."[1]

Where do you want to go in your life? Who do you want to become? What kind of life do you want to live? Do you envision a life full of energy to fulfill your goals? Or do you see one that's physically broken down with little motivation to conquer your dreams? Set your sight on a "life vision," not on your current desire to lose weight.

Depending on your circumstances, you may have lost sight of the vision you once had. There was a season in my life where I found it difficult to dream for my future. My circumstances put a blanket over my hopes and aspirations, and I found it difficult to uncover the plans God had for me. I lacked the strength to see much beyond the present moment. Yet as I allowed Him to walk me through that season of healing, I started to dream again and believe the promises that He had for my life. I thought I had lost *me* through the years of pain, but I wasn't lost to God. He knew exactly where I was; He was there to rescue me. He was there to heal me, to restore me, and to fulfill His plans and purposes in my life.

Below is a general overview for my life that encircles what is important to me. I want to:

* feel good physically
* have energy to keep up with my awesome teenagers
* be an engaged parent
* grow old gracefully

- have the stamina to travel and be active
- avoid unnecessary doctor's visits, illnesses and diseases
- have a clear mind
- love fully
- give abundantly
- work hard
- be prepared to walk in God's plans for my life
- laugh abundantly
- cry with honesty
- face my fears
- share the wisdom I have learned
- teach others
- have fun

All this won't be possible if I'm unhealthy, overweight, tired and numb. The vision for my life reaches further than the physical change of losing weight. The goals for my life are rooted in the one who loves me unconditionally and holds dreams for me that are more magnificent than I can fathom. And oh, how I welcome the revelation of my life-adventure with God!

JOURNAL

What kind of life do you envision for yourself? Let the bigger vision drive your physical transformation. Don't let the cycle of losing weight drive your emotional and spiritual life.

Now is the time to be honest with yourself and assess how much the desire and goal to lose weight has driven the rest of your existence. How much of your emotional life have you invested in the dieting process? How many of your thoughts have been centered on food and dieting? Instead, make the larger vision for your life be the passion that consumes your time, energy, thoughts and emotions.

Envision the life you yearn to live, and let that image be the motivation for nurturing your physical body. Don't let losing weight become the catalyst that drives your actions. Let your purpose drive your health and weight loss dreams. Instead of fixating your thoughts on a number on the scale, or visualizing how you would look in a bathing suit, set your focus on the greater vision for your life. Your desire for physical change will now flow out of the entirety of who you are and your God-given purpose, rather than from the singular objective to lose weight.

Pray about the vision God holds for your life regarding your family, finances, fun and spiritual, emotional and physical health. Write down a vision statement, and then expand that statement as you dream of the life you want to live and the legacy you want to leave behind.

Dream big! Don't limit yourself by saying, "Oh, that sounds ridiculous." Maybe it's too late to be a ballerina; but no matter how old you are, you can always learn to dance! Don't let your life circumstances choke out the dreams of your youth. God still has a plan for your life even if you have taken a detour along the way. Dare to dream big!

1. Write a vision statement that provides an overview of the life you envision for yourself.
2. Now write more specific goals including the following categories: financial, family, adventure/fun, spiritual, emotional and physical.

One of my goals is that I want to participate in the Avon two-day walk for breast cancer. That event will help me achieve a physical and adventure goal. Meanwhile, a family goal that's important to me is taking a vacation with my husband and four kids each year. My emotional goals are not linked to a grand dream, but involve small choices that will maintain my emotional health, like nurturing good friendships with lunch dates or taking walks together.

The idea here is to dream! Write them down so that when the busyness, hardships or circumstances of life begin to blanket your dreams, you can remind yourself of the ones yet to be accomplished.

On a personal note, I'm still working on creating my life goals. I'm learning to dream big with God again. I will say it's exciting to see God renew the dreams I thought had been buried long ago, and to see Him birth new ones as well. If you've found it difficult to dream lately, I encourage you to give yourself permission to do so. It isn't too late to see forgotten dreams re-birthed or new dreams born. Put your doubts and fears to the side and dream!

Alignment Questions: What am I aligning myself with, and is it producing the kind of fruit I want in my life? Are you aligning yourself with a vision bigger than weight loss, or are you settling for a heavy pack of to-dos?

THOUGHTS TO PONDER AS YOU JOURNAL

1. Take stock of your current health, and use the symbolism of furniture and décor to describe it. What do you hope for it to look like?
2. Has taking care of your health been similar to lugging a heavy backpack?
3. Do you believe your health can be a byproduct of who you are instead of a to-do list to accomplish? What does that look like?
4. What reasons motivate you to lose weight?
5. Name other motivations beyond the goal of weight loss.
6. Describe the bigger life vision you can use to replace your shortsighted goal of weight loss.
7. How have you let the hardships of life diminish your capacity to dream?
8. Allow yourself to dream without filtering. Write down what you discover.

RECOMMENDED READING FOR WEEK SIX
The Circle Maker: Praying Circles Around Your Biggest Dreams and Greatest Fears by Mark Batterson

JOURNAL NOTES

Week Seven

~~~

CHAPTER 13

OPENING YOUR GIFTS

IF WE CHOOSE TO SEE our health as a tedious checklist to complete on a daily basis, we will continue to feel discouraged with what remains on the list. If we're going to change our mindset from to-do lists to a life vision, we'll need to view our health from a different perspective.

Let's imagine that someone very special to you has given you a beautifully wrapped gift. You know this person pays careful attention to detail when picking a present, and you anticipate the perfect gift. Do you rush to open it, or do you casually set it on the counter to ponder what is inside? I imagine you would eagerly open the present with excited anticipation of what it contains. I know I would.

Referring again to the analogy of our health being a room in a house, God has given us many gifts to fill that space. Do we set His gifts – unopened – on the table in a dingy room that lacks life and luster, or do we open them and begin to decorate?

As God's gifts are opened and placed in our old, unhealthy room, they bring brightness: a ray of sunshine that fills the room. We can see the cobwebs that formed due to neglect, enabling us to sweep them away. We recognize that the furniture is drab and worn out, so we invest in new furniture that matches our personality: sporty, causal, contemporary. We fill our room with treasures, allowing nothing that's second rate.

If we never open our gifts, this area will be filled with packages, yet remain dingy and unappealing. Our health room can be filled with light and beauty. But all too often, due to neglect and discouragement, it becomes a place we avoid. It's dark, sad and in desperate need of a breath of life.

Do we see our health journey as a gift, or do we view it as the weighted backpack of to-dos? God has given us the precious gifts to redecorate and transform our physical beings. Let's begin by opening His gifts.

Your Body Is a Valuable Gift from God

You may look in the mirror and have difficulty viewing your body as a gift in and of itself. But you are so precious to God. He not only made you with the greatest of care, but He also made you to be where His Holy Spirit dwells; your body is His temple (1Corinthians 3:16, 6:19).

Pause for a moment and let that thought sink in for a moment. My first instinct is to question why in the world God would decide to do that. The answer: Because He loves us! We are His children, and His Spirit is His promise to us (Ephesians 1:13-14).

Your body is designed most intricately. I understand little about the human body and how it works, but in my limited knowledge, I can grasp how cool it is. For example, when we cut ourselves, the body naturally clots so we don't bleed to death; and limbs that are broken produce new cells and blood vessels to rebuild the bone.[1]

The body is designed to heal and care for itself. The way we treat it determines whether it can keep up with that process. If we poorly nourish our body, over time, it will lack the ability to restore the damage that has been done. The result: We begin to experience health issues such as high cholesterol, high blood pressure, diabetes and heart disease. On the other side of the spectrum, health enthusiasts have claimed for years that consuming certain foods can prevent and even reverse many of these conditions. Science is now beginning to provide the proof that supports these claims.

The bottom line is that our bodies are truly a gift from God. Do you see yours as a gift or a disappointment?

Fruits and Veggies Are Gifts of Medicine to Your Body

When we value food – not as a list of "can't haves," but as a gift that enables us to pursue our purpose in life – then we'll develop a different attitude and a healthier relationship with it. We'll begin to appreciate its life-giving benefits rather than focusing on feeling deprived.

Food was not created to tease and taunt us, but rather to be peacefully enjoyed. Food, in its natural state, was created to fuel our bodies with life sustaining energy. Fruits and vegetables are natural foods that God created to promote health, strength, endurance and life.[2] He gave us "every seed-bearing plant on the face of the whole earth and every tree that has fruit with seed in it" (Genesis 1:29 NIV). These nutrients help rebuild our cells, keeping sickness and disease at bay.[3] They are cleansing foods that are alkaline-forming and help eliminate impurities by removing toxins from the body.[4]

When you research the nutrients in fruits and vegetables and their essential role, it's amazing to discover how they serve as powerful medicine for our bodies. When we investigate the nutritional value of strawberries, we learn that they contain vitamin C, calcium, magnesium and fiber. They help to lower cholesterol, reduce the risk of heart disease and help fight inflammation.[5] One simple berry contains a powerful medicinal impact. Our food is a wonderful gift that we should open and cherish daily. It acts as medicine to maintain health and heal the body.

And don't forget the other nutritional gifts like whole grains, which help aid digestion, and lower cholesterol and blood pressure.[6] Good fats reduce the risk of heart disease, and lean protein helps to regulate blood sugar and build muscle.[7] Whole foods, in their natural state, provide nutrients that enhance health and promote healing. Food was not meant to be toxic, promoting sickness and disease. God's gifts are pure and simple.

How do you view healthy food: as time consuming, inconvenient and expensive, or as a gift?

WATER AS A GIFT

We've been told to drink at least eight glasses of water a day, but do we really understand why? It's not simply a technique to help us lose weight and insure that we run to the bathroom every hour. Our bodies are made of approximately 60% water.[8] This natural liquid delivers nutrients to our cells and is essential for flushing toxins out of the body. We can't live without it. If our bodies are deprived of it for three to five days, they begin to shut down and then death is right around the corner. Three to five days!

Do we complain over the chore of drinking water, or do we value it as a precious gift of life?

EXERCISE IS A GIFT – NOT A CURSE

I realize that exercise, for some, is a four-letter word: a dreaded part of the dieting process. Imagine yourself holding a beautifully wrapped gift that, upon opening, will provide the following:

- Improved sleep
- Stronger heart muscles
- Reduced bad cholesterol
- Toned muscles
- Improved circulation
- Increased energy levels
- Reduced stress levels
- Less addictive cravings
- Reduced risk of heart disease
- Better digestion
- Improved posture
- Improved mood
- Retarded premature aging
- Decreased blood pressure
- An added aid in weight loss
- Decreased arthritis symptoms
- Elevated metabolism
- Relieved menopausal symptoms
- Improved complexion
- Boosted self-confidence[9, 10]

Would you open that gift? The act of exercise should be approached in the same manner as any other activity that maintains the physical body, such as brushing our teeth, taking a shower or sleeping. We complete these tasks to preserve our physical body. We wouldn't envision letting our teeth rot from not brushing. So why is exercise any different? Why do we find it acceptable for our body to atrophy from lack of exercise?

Exercise is the gift I'm learning to open on a regular basis as part of my physical maintenance routine. I've realized that, to live the life God has planned for me, exercise is not an option. Being tired after a long day of work or having a busy schedule are no longer valid excuses.

Why Is Your Health Optional?

As Americans, we are first-rate pill takers. If the doctor prescribes a medication for an ailment, we fill the prescription and swallow the pill without giving it much thought. But what if, instead of just taking a pill, we took the necessary steps to make our health a priority rather than an option?

My sweet mom was overweight much of her life and found it difficult to stay committed to a healthy lifestyle. She suffered from conditions associated with obesity and took numerous medications to treat them. She became diabetic in her early thirties; and as a result, she also had high cholesterol, high blood pressure and heart disease, which required multiple surgeries to treat. She passed away at the age of 72 when her body decided it couldn't take any more. My mom was a diligent pill taker. If the doctor said "take this pill," she obeyed. But what if she had instead understood how beautifully her body was made and that maintaining her health was not optional? She still may have lived a life with sickness, but the quality of her life would have been greatly impacted by consistently opening the gifts of healthy food and exercise.

There are many daily tasks that are completed as part of the routine maintenance of caring for a home, like washing dishes or doing laundry. Imagine ignoring your dirty dishes for several days or weeks, then visualize the hardened decay of food on them. Our bodies, when ignored for months or even years, will also decay, becoming toxic and sick. If the thought of rotten food from forgotten dishes makes us wince, then why do we accept the decay of our bodies as normal or expected?

When we wash the dishes, we may not get excited about the process. (I know I don't.) But we do it anyway so that our house remains warm, inviting and maintained. This simple daily act adds up to the *greater goal* of creating a home. Taking routine care of our health is part of a *greater goal* beyond just physical maintenance; it plays a significant role in creating a life full of passion and vision.

Some health-related tasks should no longer be considered optional, but regarded as necessary elements to take proper care of the house God has provided. Remember your health room. Even if it is dingy and old, a little daily care can restore its luster and life.

Open the gifts of health on a daily basis to nourish your body, not as a to-do list but as an essential part of living. The daily actions that you take add up to a lifetime of health. Your body is so precious; and with simple maintenance, it will remain in peak condition with less complications and breakdowns. Instead of focusing on the duty of eating healthy and exercising, open these gifts God provided as a rewarding part of your daily routine.

JOURNAL

I want you to create a mental picture of what your health room looks like when decorated by God's knowledge. What does your room look like when it's filled with the precious and pleasant riches of healthy foods, water and exercise? Write down what you see. What does this gift of health look like for you? How will it feel? How do *you* feel?

Now that you have a picture of what your health can look like, ask God to reveal the "spirit of your mind" – the negative attitudes that need to be renewed towards your body, healthy foods and exercise (Ephesians 4:23).

For example, do you think and speak about these things as gifts, or rather as curses or punishments? Do you moan and murmur about exercise? Do you complain that healthy foods are more expensive and time-consuming? Do you look in the mirror and pinpoint all the features of your body that you dislike?

Write down where you have adopted a negative outlook toward the gifts of knowledge that God has provided. Ask Him to forgive you for murmuring and complaining, and to renew your mind and attitude toward His precious gifts of health. (Philippians 2:14).

For those of you who are visual learners, I want you to wrap a small gift. Place the present within sight as a reminder of the gift of health that God has provided. As you open your gifts of nutritious food and exercise daily, let God's love permeate every nook and cranny of your precious health and fill your room with abundant treasures.

Alignment Questions: What am I aligning myself with, and is it producing the kind of fruit I want in my life? Do I align myself with a to-do list and an attitude that my health is a chore? Or do I celebrate the gifts God has given me?

THOUGHTS TO PONDER AS YOU JOURNAL

1. What is your attitude towards the gifts of healthy food and exercise?
2. What are the reasons you have allowed your health to be optional?
3. Taking care of your health is part of a greater goal beyond weight loss. Describe the longer-lasting goal that is your motivation for taking care of your health.
4. Describe how your body is a gift.

RECOMMENDED READING FOR WEEK SEVEN
Greater Health God's Way-7 Steps to Inner and Outer Beauty by Stormie Omartian

JOURNAL NOTES

_____

_____

_____

_____

_____

_____

_____

_____

_____

_____

_____

_____

_____

_____

_____

_____

_____

_____

_____

_____

_____

_____

_____

_____

_____

_____

_____

_____

Week Eight

CHAPTER 14

~♪

HEALTHY EATING GUIDELINES

STOP!!!

If you've jumped ahead and skipped the first two-thirds of this book, go back and read from the beginning. I know from my own experience that, when I bought a new diet or health book, the first place I would flip to would be the "eating plan." I would read it first and then eventually get around to reading the rest. Maybe.

If you forgo reading the first part of *The Lost Weight Workshop*, this experience will be an epic fail. Guaranteed! The purpose of this book is different from the other ones you have read. Discovering the truths about the dieting process and who you are is essential to your success. So turn to Week One instead. Take time with each section. Journal, question, explore, listen and seek truth. Relish the process of discovery, not the thrill of losing weight. For those of you who actually read Weeks One-Seven, continue reading. If that's not you, flip back to the beginning and enjoy digging into all that God has for you.

What you read below will not be some invention of the latest and greatest method to lose weight and transform your body. You won't find any before-and-after pictures with six-pack abs and total body makeovers. I'm not reinventing the wheel when it comes to weight loss.

When we choose a diet, we normally seek a plan that tells us exactly what to eat, when to eat it and in what quantity. But let's be honest: Most of us already know the what, how and when. We may be a little confused by all the "health information" out there: "Should I eat carbs? Should I eat after 6 p.m.? Should I eat a lot of protein, a little protein, fat or no fat?" But when we let the confusion settle, the "plan" is simple. The basis for any set of eating guidelines consists of Basic Nutrition 101: Eat fruits and vegetables, lean protein, whole grains, low-fat dairy and healthy fat. The goal is to eat more nutrient-dense foods and less empty-calorie foods.

I apologize that it isn't more exciting than that, but we now know that the real plan is not the food we eat, but the relationship we have with the food we consume. Our goal is lasting peace with the dieting process, a healthy relationship with all food, a love for ourselves, and the ability to rest in God's affection and promises. The plan is birthed from the way in which we decide to walk out our vision for life, not merely a desired goal to lose weight.

Let's begin with opening the gifts.

Eat plenty of leafy greens, other vegetables and fruit by filling your plate with an ample amount of fruit and vegetables with each meal.

Eat lean protein and non-meat protein. (e.g., chicken, fish, lean beef, tofu, eggs, Greek yogurt, protein powder). One tip is to eat a small portion of protein with each meal and snack to help keep you satisfied (e.g., an apple with peanut butter, fruit with Greek yogurt, vegetables with hummus, protein powder in smoothies).

Begin replacing white-flour products with whole-grain flour products. This does not mean you'll never again eat delicious, white bread. You may eat white-flour products. Remember: All foods are permissible. The goal is not denial or elimination; the goal is to more often than not choose a healthier replacement.

When you do, you'll discover that, as you begin eating more nutrient-dense foods, your taste buds will desire healthier options. You won't crave the white flour, processed foods. Now, again, this is a guideline. If the thought of replacing your regular pasta noodles with the whole wheat version makes you weep like a baby, then eat your pasta and enjoy! Over time, you'll discover other ways to incorporate whole grains into your eating plan.

Begin to replace white sugar and artificial sweeteners with raw honey, maple syrup or stevia. I enjoy a sweet treat, and I realize that sugar can still be a part of my healthy lifestyle if I feed my body nutrient-rich foods. When the ratio of healthy foods and sugar becomes unbalanced, I begin the cycle of increased cravings, which ultimately leads to eating more sugar and less nutrient-dense food. That cycle isn't easy to break because my body no longer desires healthy foods; it just wants the rich, sugary substitutes. To ensure I maintain this balance, I now focus on living a life of vision and passion, which far outweighs the immediate pleasure of overindulging in treats.

Also, don't be fooled into thinking you're doing yourself a favor with artificial sweeteners. True, they have fewer calories than natural sugars like honey. But is saving a mere 30 calories worth the sacrifice to your health? Be a wise consumer and do your research. Bless your body with God's natural sugars and not a manmade substitute.

Raise your glasses high and drink up (water, of course). Remember: Water is a part of your daily gifts to be opened.

Schedule exercise three times a week or more. The key word is "schedule!" To redesign our old, musty health room into a clean, inviting space, exercise is no longer optional. When you wake in the morning, you may not necessarily feel like going to work, but you still go. Regularly choosing not to would yield serious negative consequences. Going, whether we like our job or not, is something we "just do." Exercise is a "just do" gift. If we wait too long to open it, we'll face serious consequences: a body that atrophies and deteriorates. In the same way, exercise is something we do whether we like it or not.

It's never too late to start an active lifestyle. No excuses. Even if you're bound to a chair, exercise in the chair. Exercise is not an option any longer. It is a gift that we open so that we can fulfill our purpose with greater impact.

Gifts come in different shapes and sizes, and so does exercise. I like to walk, not run; I enjoy dance-style exercise like Zumba rather than high-intensity workouts. In your case, uncover what brings you pleasure and do it. If you enjoy the camaraderie of group exercise, and have the necessary time and resources, join a gym or recruit a friend to workout. If not, march around your house, or do squats when getting your laundry out of the dryer. It doesn't matter what form exercise takes; the key is to schedule it and just do it! And maybe – just maybe – you'll enjoy it. What I do guarantee is that you'll benefit from the redesign of your health room while enjoying the acquisition of increased energy and vitality.

WORKING IT OUT

Below are some basic guidelines to opening the gifts of health. I've incorporated some of what I do, to "work it out" on a daily basis. Not every day will look like the example provided. I wish I could say every day looks like this for me, but it doesn't. I'm still a work in progress.

This is a journey with highs and lows, not a program to follow to perfection. The temptation will be to follow this approach as a diet plan. But don't do it! It is not a diet. If you like what I've shared, give it a try; if it doesn't fit, take it and modify it to meet your needs. You have the freedom to choose what works for you. If you have a hankering for a dip of ice cream mid-afternoon, than eat it. If breakfast sounds good for dinner or dinner suits your fancy in the morning, then you are free to switch things around.

Remember, an eating plan is just that: a plan, not a set of rules. It can be modified and changed to fit each individual need. It's just a guide, not a secret formula that will create the body of your dreams. Think of it instead as an approach to aid you in transitioning your health from an old, dingy room to a space filled with precious gifts of health. Create the plan that works for you!

If you decide to choose an eating plan from an established book or program, I encourage you to do the following:

Take inventory of how strongly you relate to the "dieter's mentality."

* Is a diet something you go on and off?
* Do you still use the terminology "cheating on my diet?"
* How is your relationship with the scale?
* If your weight goes up, do you "punish" the scale by eating or binging?
* Do you associate dieting with depriving yourself, therefore engaging the emotional battle to eat or not to eat?
* Do you experience waves of guilt or condemnation when you eat something that's not on your diet?
* Are you magnetically pulled to food because you believe you can't have it?

If you determine that you still actively operate in this mentality, I firmly recommend you continue to work on developing a peaceful relationship with food, eating and yourself. Go back to Weeks One-Seven. Soak in the newness of what God has for you. Keep asking Him to renew "the spirit of your mind" (Ephesians 4:23). Be transformed, not by the diet, but by the power of God's love.

If you determine that your "dieter's mentality" is not high and you want to follow a structured eating plan, then ask yourself, "Can I eat this way, or at least a modified version of it, for the rest of my life?" If you can't see yourself incorporating this plan into your lifestyle, then you would be better off not following it. Pick a plan that you can stick with long-term, beyond just the quick fix of weight loss.

THREE BASIC PRINCIPLES I HAVE FOUND HELPFUL TO MAINTAINING PEACE WITH FOOD:

1.   Eat every two to three hours.

If you find yourself aimlessly roaming the kitchen, seeking food or grabbing for a handful of snacks, you can choose to walk away since you know that you'll be eating within the next hour or two. Then when it is time to eat, you'll search for what you really want, which leads to the second principle...

2.   Eat what you want, making all foods acceptable.

If you don't, you'll be more drawn to what is deemed unacceptable and will eat in excess. When all foods are permitted, you're free to decide whether you really want that item or not. Most times, you'll find yourself passing right by your initial desire and selecting a healthier option. You're at peace because you know, if you don't eat ice cream or nachos today, they will be there tomorrow. You don't have to feel compelled to eat it because you know you can have it another time; it isn't forbidden.

3.   Pick a designated time to stop eating.

I have found that setting a designated time to stop eating for the day significantly helps me in maintaining a peaceful relationship with food. The evening hours are usually my time to munch. Now, instead of grazing up until bedtime – thereby taxing my digestive system – I stop at 7:00 p.m. (This is not a hard-and-fast rule, just a guideline). I am free to eat what I want throughout the day, yet I end up eating less altogether. You may find following this habit helpful as well.

My Sample Plan

In the Morning:

I start most days with a smoothie that's jam-packed with nutrients. I view this as medicine for my body, like a pill that the doctor has prescribed to prevent disease. It has become as routine as taking my daily vitamins. I simply don't give it a second thought; I just drink it! I love that I can pack so many nutrient-dense foods into one smoothie that wouldn't necessarily taste good otherwise, because the flavors are camouflaged by the other delicious ingredients.

Smoothie base:

* One cup of water; or for a creamier texture, use milk (low-fat, almond, rice, soy) or Greek yogurt
* A handful of greens (kale, baby spinach or a mix)
* Frozen fruit of choice (strawberries, blueberries, banana for sweetness)
* Packet of stevia; or for a treat, a teaspoon of raw honey

Add-ins:

* Protein powder of choice (organic rice, hemp or whey)
* Healthy oil (3-6-9 oil, coconut oil, flax seed or chia seeds)
* Teaspoon of oat bran
* Touch of cinnamon
* Chunk of raw ginger
* Half a small raw beet, or a quarter of a large one

This smoothie, like medicine, feeds the body with vitamins, minerals and disease-fighting phytochemicals that help reduce levels of cholesterol, lower blood pressure, decrease inflammation, reduce cancer risk, fight against memory loss and diminish the risk of cardiovascular disease.[1] Now you know why I call it a medicine smoothie. So much goodness in one drink!

If you want to try drinking a nutrient-packed smoothie and this is all new to you, simply start with the standard base and add additional, nutrient-rich foods over time. Research some healthy smoothie ingredients, and you may discover your own favorite recipe.

Tip: A standard blender may not pulverize all the ingredients, which will result in a chunky mixture. I prefer a smooth consistency, so I use the economical, personal-size Ninja blender, but I also have friends that recommend the NutriBullet. And there are other similar models on the market that work well for grinding everything up smoothly. Please don't feel that you have to spend several hundred dollars on a high-power blender. Those are nice; but for daily use, the smaller, personal-size options have a powerful motor to effectively work.

My day is fashioned for success when I start by drinking my smoothie. I find that I don't continually crave sugar, I'm not roaming the kitchen at night searching for something to eat, and I make better choices throughout the day. During one holiday season, I stopped drinking my smoothie, and some old habits returned. My sugar intake increased, and I was never really satisfied after I ate. I've decided that feeding my body this shot of medicine is worth the effort to achieving the life I envision.

MID-MORNING SNACK IDEAS:

- Ezekiel bread toasted with fruit spread
- Apple with natural peanut butter and raw honey
- Greek yogurt with walnuts
- Healthy granola bar

LUNCH:

* Salad with some type of lean protein of choice (tuna, chicken, veggie burger, turkey)
* Homemade soup
* Sandwich on whole-grain bread with fruit or cut-up veggies

AFTERNOON SNACK IDEAS (IN ADDITION TO THE MID-MORNING SNACK):

* One of my favorites: hummus with feta cheese and cherry tomatoes
* Green smoothie
* Popcorn or a healthier variety of tortilla chip with salsa

DINNER:

Dinner, I find more challenging to prepare healthy meals for my family, mainly due to time and planning ahead. Honestly, the evening meal can be fairly lame at our house: too many nights of boxed macaroni and cheese and bowls of cereal. (Like I said, I'm still a work in progress.) When I do cook, I keep it quick and easy.

* Pasta
* Chicken or beef, throw in a vegetable and a potato or noodle, and voila! It's dinner
* Pizza on Friday, fix a salad and enjoy a piece of pizza
* Leftover night, eat leftovers or make a veggie burger on a sprouted grain bun and add a salad or cup of soup

If I just don't want to bother, I make a smoothie with fruits, veggies, and Greek yogurt or a scoop of protein powder. It's quick and nutritious.

Dessert:

* Gingersnaps
* Dip of ice cream (I use a cone so I don't unconsciously overindulge)
* A fruit smoothie made with frozen bananas, almond milk, cinnamon and raw honey (it is thick and creamy with a texture like soft ice cream... Yum!)

Remember: You can still enjoy a sweet treat. The goal is to be at peace with all food. When we choose to enjoy empty-calorie foods, we can do so without guilt.

My intention with the previous "Working It Out" section is to share some ideas and tips that work for me. As I said, if you like what I have shared, then give it a try. If not, modify it or completely revamp it with your own plan that fits your lifestyle.

THOUGHTS TO PONDER AS YOU JOURNAL

1. An eating plan is just a plan. What should it look like so you can peacefully live with it for the rest of your life?
2. If you were disappointed with the simplicity of the eating plan in Week Eight, what were you looking for? Why do you keep looking for the next best thing when eating healthy is a simple, common-sense approach?

JOURNAL NOTES

_____

_____

_____

_____

_____

_____

_____

_____

_____

_____

_____

_____

_____

_____

_____

_____

_____

_____

_____

_____

_____

_____

_____

_____

_____

_____

_____

CHAPTER 15

Getting off Track

WHAT HAPPENS WHEN WE FIND ourselves getting off track? For a season, we have maintained a healthy eating and exercise routine; we're at peace with the process, and all is well. But then our journey begins to veer off course. It may be a sudden crash that brings us to a standstill, or it may be several wrong turns that lead to an undesired destination. The sudden crash may be a night or more of binging propelled by an emotional reaction, or we may make small, unhealthy choices that lead to former patterns and a lifestyle we thought we escaped. The issue is not whether we'll get off course; life is messy, and from time to time, we'll find ourselves astray. The question is how we'll handle it when we suddenly find ourselves adrift from the healthy life we intended.

One afternoon, my husband and I were engaged in a conversation of a serious nature. I left the discussion with a flood of emotions. I wasn't sure of everything I was feeling, but they were coming hard and fast. Earlier that day, my eating had been hit or miss. It started with my medicine smoothie, but after church, we ordered pizza. I was really hungry, so instead of eating one piece and a salad, I chose two slices. And then I found myself snacking all afternoon because my body wasn't satisfied.

Later that evening, I wanted to eat and I wasn't looking to eat a piece of broccoli. I knew my desires weren't based on actual hunger but on emotions I didn't understand how to process. I was tired and I lacked the energy or desire to discover what I was feeling, so instead, I chose food.

So yes, I veered off course that day. But more significant was how I reacted afterwards. Did I continue to eat food to mask the emotional pain? Did I heap on guilt and condemnation? Did I allow anxiety to rise, fearing I would lose control?

No, the very next morning – even though I didn't feel like it – I made a conscious decision to drink my medicine smoothie.

The emotions that arose following the conversation with my husband didn't magically disappear the next morning. But instead of turning to food, I started a conversation with God, attempting to understand and decipher what I was feeling, whether anger, betrayal, sadness, etc. My heart issues didn't go away, but my response changed. Food was not meeting my emotional needs that day. It was a new day, with fresh mercies for that day, and I had a choice to walk in the newness or walk in the old ways of numbing my heart.

This is important. If we've operated in the dieting system for some time, our natural response when we use food to fill our emotional cravings is to beat ourselves up, piling on the guilt and condemnation. In response to the emotional distress, we operate in our defeated belief system, enabling the pattern of turning to food for comfort to continue. But we can stop the cycle!

We do have a choice. We are no longer bound by our old outlet of abusing food, and we're not stuck on the emotional rollercoaster that keeps taking us off course. We have put off the old self (Ephesians 4:22-24 NIV). We do have a choice: to put on the new man that understands the depth of God's love and believes the promises of God, allowing these truths to steer us back on course. It's not out of striving that we break the cycle, but out of accepting the reality of who we are in Christ.

God has a plan for you, and that plan includes freedom from the bondage to food and dieting. That is your truth! If you hear yourself making excuses, saying, "Yeah, but…," then go back and soak in the love of God. Read His word and ask Him to make it real to you. Then thank God for the person He created you to be and for His promises. Allow yourself the freedom to joyously thank Him. Get excited about your life and the plans He holds for you.

It's hard for the downhill cycle of dieting to prevail when you push it aside with the joy that comes from knowing God's promises. Don't walk another day in the defeated belief system that you're not worthy, or that you won't be able to have a healthy relationship with food, and be successful at losing weight! Walk in the truth of what God says about you.

You have the victory. Make the choice to believe.

Alignment Questions: What am I aligning myself with: a defeated dieter's belief system, or the voice of victory and hope? Is it producing the type of fruit I want in my life?

THOUGHTS TO PONDER AS YOU JOURNAL

1. What is your immediate response when you find yourself off track with your eating plan?
2. What choices can you make to redirect your path when you veer off course?

JOURNAL NOTES

_____

_____

_____

_____

_____

_____

_____

_____

_____

_____

_____

_____

_____

_____

_____

_____

_____

_____

_____

_____

_____

_____

_____

_____

_____

~

CHAPTER 16

Putting It All Together

How do we apply the knowledge gained from *The Lost Weight Workshop* on a day-to-day basis? I could compile a list of helpful hints to guide you through this journey. If I did, it might look a lot like this:

- Be completely present when you eat
- Eat on a smaller plate
- Put your utensils down between bites
- Drink a glass of water before you eat
- Don't eat carbs with the evening meal
- Write down everything you eat
- Plan your meals
- Cook meals for the week on the weekends
- Clean out your food pantry and restock with healthy foods
- Cut up veggies and keep them in the fridge

All of these tips can be beneficial in the weight loss journey, but most of us already know these and more. If we're not careful, these tips become a strict set of rules to follow.

The LWW principles are not based on a "to-do list," but rather an experience that's walked out on a daily basis. These truths are a **"TODAY**

Experience," not something we wish or dream for tomorrow, but something for **now**!

Below, you'll find the Lost Weight Workshop "TODAY Experience" declaration. Write these statements down on a piece of paper or copy the declaration from Appendix B. Put it where you can see it each morning: on the bathroom mirror, in your Bible, on the refrigerator. Proclaim the following statements as your decree that your health will be a "TODAY Experience!"

DECLARE BOLDLY:

Today, dieting is not the answer to losing weight. God holds the answer.

Today, when I look in the mirror, I will not focus on what I look like, but I will choose to speak God's truth that I am fearfully and wonderfully made.

Today, if life seems to be pressing down, I will confess the bigness of God and His word into my circumstances.

Today, if I am consumed with thoughts of food and dieting, I will refocus on the greater vision of my life.

Today, if I am emotionally eating, I will ask the question "what am I feeding?"

Today, I will open the gifts of health and exercise as an essential part of my life rather than as an option.

Today, I renew my attitude and put off the former self by having a heart of thanksgiving and praise.

Instead of moving through each day guided by a weary checklist, the principles of the LWW will carry you, flowing from the inside out: from who you are. You are in the process of renewing your mind, emotions and spirit. You may have operated in the old dieting pattern for many years, making it second nature to breathing. But you're learning to do this diet thing differently, so have patience. Keep soaking in the truth of God's Word and the principles laid out in the LWW as He leads you through this wonderful transformation.

The Lost Weight Workshop is a today experience – *a today experience* of love, of healing, of transformation and of freedom; not a *today experience* of perfection, of guilt, of self-hatred and of bondage. Which will you choose?

Journal
Make a copy of the "Today Experience" Declaration located in Appendix B. Read and proclaim it daily.

JOURNAL NOTES

_____

_____

_____

_____

_____

_____

_____

_____

_____

_____

_____

_____

_____

_____

_____

_____

_____

_____

_____

_____

_____

_____

_____

_____

_____

_____

_____

_____

_____

CLOSING THOUGHTS

You have completed reading *The Lost Weight Workshop*, but your journey is far from over. Because the LWW is a day-to-day journey, you will have a lifetime of todays that will create a future built on peace and freedom from the reliance on food and dieting. Each day, you will be faced with a choice: a choice to align yourself with a dieting system that promotes a high failure rate, an unhealthy relationship with food, and an emotional roller coaster of guilt, condemnation and anxiety... or to wholeheartedly follow a path that ends in victory, peace with food and a vision-filled life. This second choice involves a journey that fills your health room with precious gifts and is founded on a love that will take you far beyond anything you ever imagined.

The choice is yours. Take back control. Don't let the diet, your emotions or your thoughts be the determining factors that govern your life. Let God's truth be your foundation: His heart, His word, His love, His life. Don't ever forget that no matter what number the scale reveals, you are a precious child of God; and nothing can ever change that fact. Nothing can ever separate you from His unfailing love (Romans 8:38-39)!

Your emotions may scream that you're unworthy; your thoughts may say that you don't measure up to the expectation of beauty. But throw all that to the wind. Those beliefs are counterfeit.

Today, build your life on the foundation of the truth of who you are in Christ, choosing to no longer accept the lies of defeat. With outstretched arms, fully seize the lavish love of your heavenly Dad. Embrace the new. Throw out the old. And, by golly, let's do this thing called dieting and weight loss differently!

Blessings,

Mama K Imhof

If reading *The Lost Weight Workshop* has made a difference in your life, please spread the word to others. Give a copy to a friend or to your church leadership, rate it on Amazon.com or share about it on social media. My prayer is that this book will find its way into the hands of those who will be blessed by its message.

Appendix A

~

Daily Tracker

THE PURPOSE OF THE TRACKER is to direct your thoughts and energy on God and His promises, rather than focusing on food and whether or not you "performed well" on your eating plan. As you read through *The Lost Weight Workshop*, it should become apparent that your success on the weight loss journey has more to do with what you believe about yourself and God, than dieting itself. Change is not measured by how well you perform on your diet, but how deeply you come to know your heavenly Dad and his promises for you. So to do that, you will want to spend time with Him, working through the journal portions of this book and using the daily tracker as a helpful tool for the process.

Using the Daily Tracker

1. Begin your day with a Scripture of your choice. I've provided a list of Scriptures divided by different needs. You can choose one that speaks directly to your heart's desire for that day.
2. As you go throughout your day, mark the gifts you open. If you didn't open as many as you planned, focus on what you did open, and don't condemn yourself for what remained. Remember: Your health is not

a heavy backpack filled with a to-do list to accomplish but rather a gift to open (as discussed in Weeks Six and Seven).

3. Ask God, did I feed my heart today? If you ate because you were bored or stressed… write it down. Then ask God to reveal if there was a deeper emotional issue that you were feeding (as discussed in Weeks Four and Five).

4. Confess God's promises into your situation. If you're eating due to life's hardships, don't enable yourself to wallow in the circumstance. Pour out your heart to God, but be like David and proclaim the bigness of your Father's love into your situation (as discussed in Week Four).

5. End your day with a heart of thanksgiving. On this journey, we can tend to focus on the negative: how we've blown it! We've overeaten. We feel fat. We didn't exercise. But let's change the "attitude of our mind" and focus on the positive. The perfect starting point is a heart of thanksgiving.

SCRIPTURES TO START YOUR DAY

SUCCESS

Psalms 37:5-6
Philippians 3:13-14
Proverbs 3:5-6
Proverbs 21:2-3
Romans 8:31-32
Proverbs 16:3

Jeremiah 29:11
Jeremiah 17:7-8
Matthew 17:20
Romans 5:3-5
1 Corinthians 10:13

NEWNESS

Romans 12:1-2
Ephesians 4:22-24
Jeremiah 1:5
Ephesians 2:10

Philippians 2:14
Psalms 139:13-14
1 Corinthians 6:19-20

PROVISION

Matthew 6:25-30
Philippians 4:19
2 Corinthians 9:8
Ephesians 3:20

Luke 12:22-23
Matthew 7:11
Matthew 6:20-21

God's Love

Isaiah 54:10
Psalm 25:10
Psalm 103:11
Psalm 33:22
John 3:16

Ephesians 3:16-19
Psalm 36:5
Psalms 118:1-4
Romans 8:38-39

Forgiveness

Psalm 86:5
Ephesians 4:32
Colossians 3:13

1 John 1:9
Isaiah 43:25

Peace

Philippians 4:6-9
Psalms 62:1-2
Isaiah 41:13
Isaiah 41:10
Psalm 4:8

Exodus 33:14
Romans 15:13
John 14:27
Deuteronomy 33:12

Strength

Psalm 31:24
Jeremiah 17:7-8
2 Timothy 1:7
Deuteronomy 31:8
Matthew 11:28-30
Psalms 46:1-3
Isaiah 41:29-31

Isaiah 41:10
James 1:2-3
Isaiah 40:31
Joshua 1:9
Isaiah 40:28-29
Psalms 62: 1-2, 5, 7
Jeremiah 31-25

God's Goodness

Mark 11:24
Jeremiah 33:3
Jeremiah 29:11-13
Deuteronomy 4:31
Psalm 84:11
Psalm 34:8

John 14:13-14
Proverbs 15:29
Deuteronomy 31:6
Psalms 121:3, 5-8
James 1:17
Joshua 1:5

Salvation

Ephesians 2:4-9
Romans 3:23-24

1 John 4:15-16
Psalm 13:5

Encouragement

Psalm 55:22
Psalm 9:9
Psalms 34:18-19
John 16:33
Psalms 13:5-6
Joshua 1:9

1 John 1:9
Psalm 130:7
Psalms 94:18-19
Lamentations 3:21-23
Ephesians 3:16-19
Psalm 92:5

Deliverance

Psalm 34:19
Psalm 91:15

Psalms 138:7-8
Psalm 32:7

Thanksgiving

Job 8:21

Psalm 68:3

Isaiah 55:12

Psalm 126:3

Psalms 106:1-2

Psalm 32:11

Isaiah 51:11

Joel 2:23

Psalm 68:35

Direction

Psalm 119:105

Psalms 31:3

Proverbs 6:22-23

Psalm 32:8

Psalms 25:4-5

Isaiah 48:17

Proverbs 4:11

Daily Tracker

Remember: God's Mercies are new each and every day!

Scripture to start my day: _____

_____

_____

Opening the gifts

Breakfast:
Fruit/Veg _____Protein_____ Grains_____

Lunch:
Fruit/Veg _____Protein_____ Grains_____

Dinner:
Fruit/Veg _____Protein_____ Grains_____

Two to three healthy snacks:
_____, _____, _____

Water:
_____, _____, _____, _____, _____, _____, _____, _____

Exercise:
_____

What am I feeding?
_____

_____

I am thankful for:
_____

_____

Appendix B

~

The "TODAY Experience" Declaration

Today, dieting is not the answer to losing weight. God holds the answer.

Today, when I look in the mirror, I will not focus on what I look like, but I will choose to speak God's truth that I am fearfully and wonderfully made.

Today, if life seems to be pressing down, I will confess the bigness of God and His word into my circumstances.

Today, if I am consumed with thoughts of food and dieting, I will refocus on the greater vision of my life.

Today, if I am emotionally eating, I will ask the question "what am I feeding?"

Today, I will open the gifts of health and exercise as an essential part of my life rather than an option.

Today, I renew my attitude and put off the former self by having a heart of thanksgiving and praise.

Chapter 1

1   *Merriam-Webster* 13 July 2015 < http://www.merriam-webster.com/>.

Chapter 2

1   Rena R. Wing, and Suzanne Phelan, "Long-term Weight Loss Maintenance 1'2'3'4'" *American Journal of Clinical Nutrition* 2005 <http://
ajcn.nutrition.org/content/82/1/222S.long>. Proceedings of a sym-
posium "Science-based Solutions to Obesity: What are the Roles of
Academia, Government, Industry, and Health Care?" Boston, MA,
10-11 March 2004 and Anaheim, CA, 2 Oct. 2004.

2   J. Levi, L. Segal, R. St. Laurent, and J. Rayburn, "The State of Obesity-
Better Policies for a Healthier America" *RWJF* (Trust for America's
Health), Sept. 2014
<http://www.rwjf.org/en/library/research/2014/09/the-state-of-obesity>.

Chapter 5

1   Stormie Omartian, *Greater Health God's Way-7 Steps to Inner and Outer
Beauty* (Eugene: Harvest House, 1996), 83-85.

Chapter 8

1   Mark Batterson, *The Circle Maker: Praying Circles around Your Biggest
Dreams and Greatest Fears* (Grand Rapids: Zondervan, 2011), 176.

Chapter 13

1   Yamini Durani, MD,"The Facts about Broken Bones," *KidsHealth* (The Nemours Foundation) 1 Oct. 2012, 13 July 2015 <<http://kidshealth.org/kid/ill_injure/aches/broken_bones.html>.

2   Omartian, 67.

3   Omartian, 72.

4   Omartian, 70.

5   Andrea Gabrick,"Nutritional Benefits of the Strawberry," *WebMD* 31 Mar. 2008, 13 July 2015 < http://www.webmd.com/diet/nutritional-benefits-of-the-strawberry>.

6   Amanda Gardner, "18 Benefits of Whole Grains," *Huffington Post Healthy Living* 1 Aug. 2014, 13 July 2015 < http://www.huffingtonpost.com/2014/08/10/whole-grains-health-benefits_n_5655022.html>.

7   Colette Bouchez, "Good Fat, Bad Fat: The Facts About Omega 3, Think All Dietary Fat Is the Same? Guess Again," *WebMD* 13July 2015 <http://www.webmd.com/women/features/omega-3-fatty-acids>.

8   Kathleen M. Zelman, MPH, RD, LD, "6 Reasons to Drink Water. It's No Magic Bullet, but the Benefits of Water Are Many," *WebMD* 8 May 2008, 13 July 2015 <http://www.webmd.com/diet/6-reasons-to-drink-water>.

9   Sophie Breene, "13 Mental Health Benefits of Exercise," *Huffington Post Healthy Living* 27 Mar. 2013, 13 July 2015 <http://www.huffingtonpost.com/2013/03/27/mental-health-benefits-exercise_n_2956099.htm>.

10   "Exercise: 7 Benefits of Regular Physical Activity," *Mayo Clinic* 5 Feb. 2014, 13 July 2015 <http://www.mayoclinic.org/>.

Chapter 14

1   "The Health Benefits of Food. Dig into the Science of Why Some Foods Can Make You Feel Better," *Joy Bauer Official Site - Nutrition and Weight-Loss Expertise You Can Trust*, 13 July 2015 <http://www.joybauer.com/>.

Works Cited

~

"Align." Def. 1. *Merriam-Webster*. Merriam-Webster. Web. 13 July 2015.

Batterson, Mark. *The Circle Maker: Praying Circles around Your Biggest Dreams and Greatest Fears*. Grand Rapids: Zondervan, 2011. Print.

Breene, Sophie. "13 Mental Health Benefits of Exercise." *Huffington Post Healthy Living*. Huffington Post, 27 Mar. 2013. Web. 13 July 2015.

Bouchez, Colette. "Good Fat, Bad Fat: The Facts About Omega 3. Think All Dietary Fat Is the Same? Guess Again." *WebMD*. WebMD. Web. 13 July 2015.

Byrne, Rhonda. *The Secret*. New York: Atria, 2006.Print.

Durani, MD, Yamini. "The Facts about Broken Bones." *KidsHealth*. The Nemours Foundation, 1 Oct. 2012. Web. 13 July 2015.

"Exercise: 7 Benefits of Regular Physical Activity." *Mayo Clinic*. Mayo Foundation for Medical Education and Research, 5 Feb. 2014. Web. 13 July 2015.

Gabrick, Andrea. "Nutritional Benefits of the Strawberry." *WebMD*. WebMD, 31 Mar. 2008. Web. 13 July 2015.

Gardner, Amanda. "18 Benefits of Whole Grains." *Huffington Post Healthy Living*. Huffington Post, 1 Aug. 2014. Web. 13 July 2015.

"The Health Benefits of Food. Dig into the Science of Why Some Foods Can Make You Feel Better." *Joy Bauer Official Site - Nutrition and Weight-Loss Expertise You Can Trust.* Joy Bauer, 2014. Web. 13 July 2015.

Levi, PhD, Jeffrey, Segal, MA, Laura, St. Laurent, Rebecca and Rayburn, MPH, Jack. "The State of Obesity-Better Policies for a Healthier America." *RWJF.* Trust for America's Health, Sept. 2014. Web. 13 July 2015.

Omartian, Stormie. *Greater Health God's Way-7 Steps to Inner and Outer Beauty.* Eugene: Harvest House, 1996. Print.

"Universe." Def. 1. *Merriam-Webster.* Merriam-Webster. Web. 13 July 2015.

Wing, Rena R., and Suzanne Phelan. "Long-term Weight Loss Maintenance 1'2'3'4'" *American Journal of Clinical Nutrition* 82: 222S-225S. 2005. Print.

Zelman, MPH, RD, LD, Kathleen M. "6 Reasons to Drink Water. It's No Magic Bullet, but the Benefits of Water Are Many." *WebMD.* WebMD, 8 May 2008. Web. 13 July 2015.

www.ingramcontent.com/pod-product-compliance
Lightning Source LLC
Chambersburg PA
CBHW062001280526
45787CB00005B/1960